KETTLEBELL WORKOUT

Your Step by Step Guide to Using Kettlebells

(The Ultimate Kettlebell Workout to Lose Weight Using Simple Techniques)

Priscilla Lapierre

Published By Jackson Denver

Priscilla Lapierre

All Rights Reserved

Kettlebell Workout: Your Step by Step Guide to Using Kettlebells (The Ultimate Kettlebell Workout to Lose Weight Using Simple Techniques)

ISBN 978-1-77485-242-2

All rights reserved. No part of this guide may be reproduced in any form without permission in writing from the publisher except in the case of brief quotations embodied in critical articles or reviews.

Legal & Disclaimer

The information contained in this book is not designed to replace or take the place of any form of medicine or professional medical advice. The information in this book has been provided for educational and entertainment purposes only.

The information contained in this book has been compiled from sources deemed reliable, and it is accurate to the best of the Author's knowledge; however, the Author cannot guarantee its accuracy and validity and cannot be held liable for any errors or omissions. Changes are periodically made to this book. You must consult your doctor or get professional medical advice before using any of the suggested remedies, techniques, or information in this book.

Upon using the information contained in this book, you agree to hold harmless the Author from and against any damages, costs, and expenses, including any legal fees potentially resulting from the application of any of the information provided by this guide. This disclaimer applies to any damages or injury caused by the use and application, whether directly or indirectly, of any advice or information presented, whether for breach of contract, tort, negligence, personal injury, criminal intent, or under any other cause of action.

You agree to accept all risks of using the information presented inside this book. You need to consult a professional medical practitioner in order to ensure you are both able and healthy enough to participate in this program.

TABLE OF CONTENTS

INTRODUCTION 1

CHAPTER 1: KETTLEBELLS AND WELL-DESIGNED STRENGTH 5

CHAPTER 2: CHEST AND HUB 11

CHAPTER 3: THE MODE TO CHOOSE A KETTLEBELL 19

CHAPTER 4: WHAT IS IMPORTANT IS THE KETTLEBELL? ... 22

CHAPTER 5: THE ESSENTIALS TECHNIQUES 43

CHAPTER 6: MINOR BODY KETTLEBELL EXERCISES 48

CHAPTER 7: IRRITABLE TRAINING 52

CHAPTER 8: 13 SOVIET KETTLEBELL MOVES 55

CHAPTER 9: HUGE MUSCLES AND KETTLEBELLS 72

CHAPTER 10: MISTAKES TO CIRCUMVENT 76

CHAPTER 11: TYPES OF KETTLEBELLS 81

CHAPTER 12: KETTLEBELL WORKOUTS FOR NEWBIE 87

CHAPTER 13: CHOOSING KETTLE BELLS 110

CHAPTER 14: BURPEES (ASSEMBLE UP TO DOING THIS WITH 2 KETTLEBELLS) 115

CHAPTER 15: THE WHOLE BODY EXERCISES OR HOLISTIC WORKOUT 129

CHAPTER 16: GENERAL KETTLEBELL ERRORS 136

CHAPTER 17: WHAT MUCH ARE YOU CAPABLE TO LIFT? 141

CHAPTER 18: A GUIDE TO KETTLEBELL AND CROSSFIT INSTRUCTION 153

CHAPTER 19: THE MOST CAPABLE SOVIET KETTLEBELL ROUTINES... 157

CHAPTER 20: THE HEART RATE 166

CHAPTER 21: WIDEN YOUR LEGS AND WARMING UP 171

CONCLUSION... 179

Introduction

Have you ever felt that an athletic, lean and healthy body is avoiding you like a plague regardless of the efforts you make to lose weight and improve your fitness? It's not a problem for everyone. Women all over the world have faced similar issues, looking for an solution. The positive side is that you don't need to be struggling anymore. The answer is here and it is now in your hands.

The popularity of kettlebells has grown and have gained a following in the modern age increasing numbers of women, just like us are turning to kettlebells for help. Women from all kinds of backgrounds have found the solution they've been seeking. Kettlebells aren't some new fitness trend; they've been in use for more than 100 years. They're simple, practical and, most importantly, they're extremely effective in helping you shed weight and develop a muscular and lean body.

Don't be enticed by diets that only fail , but also make you feel depleted, hungry and exhausted. Let go of the notion that you need to work out for hours at the gym each day in order to maintain the body you desire. Prepare to take on fitness, health and a powerful burning of calories that melts away fat and leave you feeling confident and strong.

The secret to the success of kettlebells is their simple design. They don't require fancy equipment or spend a fortune to started. All you require to begin is a kettlebell, and you're on the journey to becoming a different you. The secret lies in not the amount you pay or the length of time you exercise. When you purchase the kettlebell, it's about how it affects the body, which makes this one piece of equipment perform for you according to how you would like it to.

It was the American Council of Exercise (ACE) has funded a research study that blew traditional exercise routines for losing fat over the head. The study published in the journal revealed that the participants who participated in the study burnt on average 272 calories in just 20 minutes. But that's not the end of it however. Participants burned an additional 6.6 energy per minute in anaerobic mode, which puts the total burn of 20 minutes at a staggering 408 calories, or 20.2 energy per minute ("New ACE Study" 2010.).

Kettlebells for Women has been written by women. As an adult woman, I realize that women need more than different approaches to males when it comes to training and weight reduction. They need it. This is the reason I've written this book with a specific purpose to meet the needs of women, their requirements, and to help women to be able to accomplish their goals and become the most perfect version of themselves they are able to be.

I'll provide you with extensive information covering all elements of the journey using kettlebells, to healthier, slimmer, and more fulfilled you.

The material included in the course is:

What are kettlebells, how they work, and the reason they're so powerful

What do you need to know before getting going and what you must know prior to beginning

How to select the kettlebell that is right for you.

How do diet and exercise can work together to bring you there

What you should know about achieving results and what results to expect

Kettlebell exercises to shed fat and tone your body

Kettlebells can be the key to success you've been searching for, but never knew you required. I'll show you how to discover how to make use of this powerful tool to meet your goals, shed weight and keep it off. So, stop dreaming of having a slimmer body and begin learning about how easy it is to achieve it using kettlebells.

Chapter 1: Kettlebells And Well-Designed Strength

A new interest in fitness is on functional training. Functional training is a set of exercises which will help you be more effective in your daily routines as well as across a variety of sports and activities , rather than focusing solely on one. Functional training is an integrated method of training that is designed to make use of all body parts in a positive way. To achieve this the practice of functional training doesn't necessarily concentrate on particular muscles as it does in traditional bodybuilding however, it instead focuses on an array of muscles during an exercise.

The style of health club training that has become popular in the last 30 years or so is an exact match to this integrative, functional method of training. The health club model employing Hammer Strength or Nautilus machines will focus on specific muscles and hypertrophy training. Although this isn't a negative way to train and may produce some impressive results if you're looking more for aesthetics but it's not the way to build strength that's as right at home in a training gym for martial arts, the yoga studio, running track or in the backyard as it is at the fitness center.

One of the main reasons to this is that training with a specific muscle group (like in a bodybuilding-style program) could distinct to a lack of awareness of other muscles, and not focusing on flexibility and mobility as part of the training program. Training that is functional takes each these aspects into consideration and seeks to combine several conflicting elements into a single, cohesive unit. How can I improve my performance at the gym to help me more effective when I go to the Muay Thai exercise center, and playing an indoor soccer match on a Friday night , and when I assist my friend to build a fence around his home on Saturday? Functional training aims to answer these kinds of questions.

Kettlebells are a functional tool for training

Kettlebell training is an excellent illustration of a functional program. Although there are instances when you'll target specific muscle groups and/or areas like presses or squats. A complete exercise and program will include various muscle groups and will result into increased calories burned and increased muscle strength and enable you to develop your body for different sports and disciplines.

A good example of this could be the swing. A simple , momentum-based exercise such as the swing involves the legs as well as the glutes, lower back shoulder, core and grip. A single movement that is also a complete body function. Research also suggests that the swing burns calories in the same way as other types exercises for endurance.

A compound exercise such as Double kettlebell thrusters is an additional example of a total body, functional exercise. The exercise will build your body's total strength and strength. Each of the smaller moves that are part of this greater exercise will help build the strength and power of the entire body.

Another reason for kettlebells being efficient in building performance are the design and the offset strength of the equipment. As a result it is possible to perform more exercises than you can by using a barbell, or your own weight. Imagine the muscle recruitment essential for a workout that consists of kettlebell squats, kettlebell goblet squats see-saw presses , and swings. It's a basic exercise, yet it permits virtually every muscle in your body to be engaged.

Kettlebells are simply the most effective tool to increase physical strength and power particularly if you have only have a tiny space or a restricted budget. Kettlebells are a great method of building strength throughout the whole body, but especially in the core and through grip. The core and grip strength are the two most crucial areas to work on since they have the best transfer into the real world needs for strength.

Stability and Mobility

One of the main functional advantages of kettlebells is the way it helps build stability and mobility, two of the fundamentals of functional fitness. Like barbells kettlebells let you make use of one arm or leg to move, but unlike dumbbells their unique shape kettlebells creates a completely different type of stimulus.

Stability and mobility are linked and are both aspects of the one coin. Mobility refers to the degree of flexibility you have - the degree to which you are in a position to move and reach an the maximum range of motion within joints. Good mobility means that you are able to bend your knees and reach your toes, or move into an squat with your feet in full extension or turn your shoulders up to ensure that your biceps are in touch with your ears, for example. Stability means using your body to to resist movements. One example of stability could being to maintain a straight back when deadlifting, or carrying the weight with one hand and resisting the urge to bend that side.

Stability and mobility are crucial indicators of overall strength and overall health. Kettlebells can help in the development of stability and mobility through the simulation of both in one move. Take the swing for an illustration. In one swing, you're increasing your mobility by the speed of the swing. You are also not rounding your back to increase stability.

While the fundamental exercises will improve the stability and mobility of your body however, more complex movements, such as the windmill, the halo and get-ups, will significantly increase your flexibility and capacity to maintain a healthy body form while moving in weakened positions.

Chapter 2: Chest And Hub

The chest and the core are crucial in the fitness world because the muscles they have are crucial in many daily tasks we perform. The chest muscles help in transmitting power to shoulders and arms, and the core is crucial because it connects the lower and upper part of your body. A weak core can impact everything from breathing to your ability to perform basic things like get up from the chair.

This chapter aims to discuss the various ways to increase your core strength and strengthen the chest muscles so that you do not only look attractive and feel great, but live the best life you can.

1. It's the Kettlebell Russian Twist

Focus muscle group: The Core (Abdominal muscles as well as Obliques)

Walkthrough The simplest and most effective exercises to build strength in the core to do can be described as an exercise known as the Russian twist. It is a classic girevoy exercise that strengthens as well as the Abdominal as well as the Oblique muscles of the core. It is among the most effective exercises to increase core strength and stability and it has been proven to do more for your core than sit-ups or crunches.

Relax your legs at an appropriate angle (less that 90 degrees) and ensure that your feet are level with the floor, approximately shoulder length apart. Lean backwards at a 45-degree angles (taking the feet of of the floor) and then turn between left and right as you are you move the kettlebell over the body, from side to the next. The movement between left and right, then back is a repetition. The recommended number of repetitions for each set is adequate, however this is yet another one of those fluid exercises you can perform in a time trial to test how long you are able to withstand the stress.

Take note also that this is an advanced version of the exercise. To ease some tension off, make sure to keep your feet off of the ground while you work out Don't be too far back.

2. It is the Kettlebell Floor Press

The target muscle group is Chest and the core

Walkthrough: This exercise is quite like a traditional dumbbell floor press, however it is quite different in several ways. The way that the weight utilized behaves is the most important because your body's response is slightly differently to the change in the center gravitational force of the load employed. A kettlebell-based floor press can be perfect for people who want to build muscles and strength in their chests. However, it also aids in the strength of your core and arm to some extent.

Similar to a traditional dumbbell press exercise, the workout starts by lying on your back , with the kettlebell in front of you. Take the kettlebell by the handle, with your palm facing towards the inside and press the weight upwards while rotating your palm. If you've done it correctly when you reach the top of the press your palm should be in front of your feet. The kettlebell should be brought back to its original position for one repetition. When you have completed the desired number of repetitions, switch hands and repeat the exercise until you do one repetition.

This workout can be performed by using two kettlebells at once in accordance with the exercise or fitness level. When using two kettlebells it is essential to have a better control over the weights since there could be the tendency to favor either hand during this workout.

3. Single Arm Kettlebell Snatch

The target muscle group is Chest

Walkthrough: The bar snatch has been in use since the same amount of time that the weightlifting industry has existed, or even longer. This amazing drill is one of the most effective ways to showcase the explosive strength of your arms and chest although the primary source of power is definitely your chest. Similar to the bar snatch exercise the primary goal for it's Single Arm Kettlebell Snatch exercise is to make your arms and the weight over your head in what appears as one continuous movement.

If you are you are snatching the kettlebell be aware that the posture is similar to that used when you do a bar snatch. It is best to stand with your legs about the same distance apart, with your knees bent, and with the kettlebell's weight on your legs. Get on your toes, and as you do this you should pull the kettlebell upwards until it is at your chest. From there, lift the weight over your head, and then lower it back to its beginning position. This is one repetition. Make sure not to hold your elbow within your body while you work the weight as you could seriously hurt yourself in the event that you do not.

4. The Kettlebell Press-up and row

Muscle group to target: Chest and Core

Guide: Man has been doing press-ups for many years. They're a crucial component of human motion, and the motion involved is the base of how a person rises from a prone posture with stomach flat on the floor. There have been a variety of variations throughout the years and all were designed to make press-ups more difficult or to exercise an additional muscle group. One thing all press-ups share is that no matter the way they're done your chest and core are working while doing them.

The main difference between kettlebell press-up and the classic press-up is the handle of the kettlebell. The smaller purchase where to place your hands makes the exercise more difficult to do with the weights. Then, when you add the variation of row it promises to be unique exercise.

Then, take your kettlebells with their handles and then get them into the traditional press-up posture. Do a traditional press-up. However, after the press-up, raise an elbow by pushing the shoulder blades together . raise the weight off of the ground by at about six inches. Lower the arm, and repeat, but this time with the other hand to carry the load. The goal is that is in between seven and five rows for each arm.

5. Single Arm Kettlebell Split Jerk

The target muscle group is Chest

Walkthrough: This is one of the most advanced girevoy exercises available and is utilized by many people to prepare for an explosive burst of muscular strength that comes from the shoulders and chest. It has been a great help to the bodybuilders of today prepare for the classic barbell jerk because it gives them better control of the weights and an effective exercise.

This is one of the exercises that is performed after a transition exercise for the first time, so cleanse the kettlebell from your shoulder while keeping your rack in place. Bend your knees and then press the kettlebell onto your head while bouncing to the split-jerk posture. While holding the weight above your head slowly pull your legs back in a way that you're back in a standing position. Bring the weight back onto the rack for one repetition.

Similar to some other one-handed kettlebell exercises, this can be completed using two hands, which adds the difficulty level to it. The added weight and the need to use two hands makes the balance challenging, adding to the overall strength you will gain from performing this exercise. It is advised to use this Double Handed Kettlebell Split Jerk only be used after it is proven that the Single Handed version has been refined to avoid injuries or strains.

Chapter 3: The Mode To Choose A Kettlebell

According to a research study by the University of Wisconsin- La Crosse There are numerous ways that you can pick the kettlebell. The kettlebells are generally different in design. Some have rubber coatings to protect floors from the impact. Others are specially designed for competitions. These kettlebells feature an elongated handle and are of uniform shape and size regardless of weight.

Through the years, a few manufacturers have created kettlebells that have a concave faces to aid in ergonomic benefits. Other kettlebells like the new-fangled kettlebells are the same as dumbbells. This means the kettlebells are able to be loaded by plates to allow weight adjustments, using just one piece of equipment. Like kettlebell swings and getups can be believed to increase the heart rate going and help burn fat similarly to how the cardio machine can, but will help in strengthening the correct mechanics.

If you are planning to purchase the kettlebell for your first time, it's crucial to perform the test before you make the purchase. Begin by putting your hand on your hands and then bringing your thumb to the top of your pinky. Note the channel that is formed in your palm. This is the spot where the handle of your kettlebell is meant to rest the majority often. It is located from the outside knuckle of the index finger and down to the opposite end of your wrist, in an arc diagonal.

Then, you can pick up the weight and holding the handle to ensure that it is able to fill the channel. Make sure that the bell rests on the forearm's back and that your wrist is straight. It is crucial to ensure that the bell does not rest on the boney shape that your forearm has. If you pull out the kettlebell

It rubs against the bone protruding from the side of your wrist that is more lateral and it rubs against the bone protruding from your wrist, this indicates that the force transfer from the hand isn't the ideal way to go about it. Also there is a significant possibility of getting injured.

The most effective safety advice to follow is to avoid selecting a kettlebell with handles that are thick. It will be apparent that Onnit's handles are diameter that is just over one inch. This is plenty for you to work your grip strength without causing fatigue.

If you are doing an exercise such as the swing, there's the possibility that you'll perform a lot of reps during a single workout. It is crucial to make sure that your grip isn't burning out. This is because it's not beneficial from a technical perspective. When your grip is stressed and the grip is overworked, it's likely that you'll experience an array of mechanical issues that can arise. In terms of how much weight you can start with, men generally lift 16 pounds, while women can manage 8 kilograms.

Chapter 4: What Is Important Is The Kettlebell?

Because the weight of a kettlebell can be adjusted it is important to know of this prior to purchasing the appropriate weight for your needs. For beginners, weights ranging from 4 and 16 kilograms are suggested for women, while women usually opt for weights with a lighter capacity of up to 10 kilograms , while men prefer heavier weights. As time passes you will gain strength and you'll be able to carry heavier weights. However, it's best to begin by using lighter weights to limit the chance of injury and make the initial phase more comfortable.

Kettlebell is a great appliance for home use. There's so many things you can accomplish with a kettlebell that will be on your mind when you read everything in one sitting. But, for now we're not here to discuss kettlebells and their benefits in general. Here are some benefits of kettlebell swings. The swing is a specific exercise that you could make like a woman using the kettlebell. Let's begin by talking about the kettlebell's advantages!

The kettlebell is possibly the most basic exercise equipment you'll ever own, but it is also among the most useful and versatile. It's a huge iron ball made of cast iron with one handle on the top. Kettlebells are used in a variety of ways and one of their most popular applications is that of the Kettlebell Swing.

What is a Kettlebell Swing?

Kettlebell Swing is a unique exercise that can be done using the kettlebell. The exercise begins with your feet and legs spaced a bit greater than shoulder width apart. The kettlebell handle is held by placing the kettlebell in between your legs. This implies that you must be able to bend your knees slightly.

Then , begin lifting the kettlebell upwards and out with your legs, core and arms to create the force required to lift the kettlebell. The final posture will be arms stretched out towards the front of you, and slightly over your head and holding the kettlebell by using straight legs. Once you've accomplished this, lower it and repeat the procedure that you did to lift it up in the first place.

Benefit 1: Receive a Total Body Workout to build Muscle

One of the greatest advantages of kettlebell swings is that they offer the complete body workout that works virtually every muscle of your body from the top to the bottom. A kettlebell swing can be an effective exercise that you can perform using the kettlebell.

In order to clarify things The first phase of the swing, where you begin swinging upwards, demands your glutes, your legs hips, hips, and lower them back down to create the force required to hold the kettlebell as it rises. When the swing is progressing and you're about to lift it, your abdominal and abdominal muscles expand to help maintain strength and strengthen your core. When you are in the upright posture of the swing your shoulders, arms lats, wings and chest muscles will work to bring them to a position that they are over your head.

As you descend you will see everything happening the opposite direction. As you can observe, a kettlebell swing can be a fantastic way to work every muscle throughout your body. The outcome of this is that you'll be able to build muscles that are stronger after a brief time.

Naturally, all of us would like more muscle mass, as they improve the performance of athletes and make life simpler and look nice. A Kettlebell Swing is a great method to get your body prepared for summer season.

Advantage 2. Kettlebell Swings are Very Versatile

Another reason which makes kettlebells swings an effective exercise is that it's extremely flexible which means everyone can master it. This exercise, as well as the kettlebell generally isn't meant exclusively for men.

Everybody, male and female both old and young can use the kettlebell. It's because the kettlebell is available in a variety of weights. Women who are smaller, elderly and children of a younger age may start out with a kettlebell that weighs less than 2.5 5, 7.5 or 10 pounds. On the other hand, middle-aged or stronger people typically have the 15, 20, 25 30 or 35 Pound kettlebells effortlessly.

They can vary in weight between 1.5 to 100 pounds or more, meaning that practically anybody can locate an appropriate kettlebell to swing the kettlebell. Additionally, you don't need to be at the gym to perform kettlebell turns.

If you have the space you can perform your own Kettlebell Swing at home, in the backyard, in the gym at the park, or even at work. Also, it is the case that buying a kettlebell will be considerably less expensive than purchasing different pieces of fitness equipment.

Advantage 3: You Can Target Certain Muscles - Different Arms

Another benefit of kettlebells is the fact that it can target a variety of muscles throughout your body. For instance, if need a great exercise that is even and consistent, as we've discussed to benefit number one, you can make use of both hands to perform this Kettlebell Swing to evenly aim towards the opposite side of your body.

But, if you want to work out one part or part of the body more side for reasons beyond your control, you can use the hand kettlebell swing in which case , they'll target the part of your body that is used to perform the turns, particularly for this specific arm.

You could even add difficulty by doing alternating the kettlebell, placing the one hand on one hand and the other one on the next, swinging the kettlebell around from one arm to another as each side changes. It's very helpful to perform an exercise such as Kettlebell Swing. Kettlebell Swing that you can pick which body parts or sides that are most focused.

Benefit 4: Swing Is Made Of more than one type of Exercise

The other major advantage that's important to mention in kettlebell turns is the ability to train various fitness elements while doing it. A heavy kettlebell requires lots of strength to move up and down repeatedly It's a kind of weight, or weight training, without a doubt.

But the kettlebell swing requires a continuous, intense motion as, with the actual kettlebell swing you will never stop moving. It is a cardiovascular component that you can do continuously you'll also work your heart.

If you are looking for an exercise to improve your endurance and strength and endurance, then the swing of the kettlebell is the best option. It's a fantastic exercise for days of cross-training, when you may want to get away from strength training, or pure cardio. A kettlebell swing can be the greatest combination of both!

Benefit 5: Training for Cardiovascular Fitness Using Kettlebells

As mentioned earlier as previously mentioned, it is said that the Kettlebell Swing is a kind of cardiovascular exercise, which means it is a workout for the heart and the muscles. If you don't believe this, simply do 20 kettlebell swings for each arm, then 20 swings with both arms. Tell us that your heart isn't getting so fast that you're afraid it's going to explode.

This exercise will increase your heart rate over your usual heart rate which is a great thing. Cardiovascular exercise is vital to your overall health and well-being.

A healthy heart lowers the chance of suffering from stroke or heart attack as well as lowers heart rates, decreases blood pressure aids in lower cholesterol levels and doesn't cause your heart to work as often and for as long as it as it continues to tick. A healthy, more robust and more efficient heart will not hinder physical performance as well.

Advantage 6: Healthier Lungs

The other benefit of kettlebells is that they to make your lungs stronger and healthier.

They also make them more efficient. Like Kettlebell Swings, you work all your muscles as well as your heart, and thus help strengthen your lungs.

It is an extremely energetic form of exercise and requires lots of oxygen in order to continue, one that places an enormous strain on your lung. The more quickly and intensely you do the Kettlebells, the more your lungs will need to be working to supply your body with oxygen needed to keep going or, more simply you can train your lungs to function more efficiently. This kind of workout allows your lungs to absorb and take in more oxygen over time. It will also make it easier for your lungs to deliver an oxygen supply to the muscles.

The end result is that your muscles are able to use increased oxygen levels available for work , which means they can be more efficient in the amount of time and effort they perform. Additionally, it is the case that you'll experience less discomfort or no pain at all down the steps or take a walk up, and the lungs that are healthy and efficient are less vulnerable to breathing-related ailments.

Kettlebell Training for Women Basic Exercise

Benefit 7: Diabetes Control

Another benefit of kettlebells is that they can go greatly in the control of your diabetes. Diabetes is caused by the body's inability to break down sugar, particularly glucose, which stays within your body and causes damage to the kidneys, liver and various organs. In the long run, this can determined to death.

But, the kettlebell swing could help in controlling this issue by eating up glucose that is not being used. Your muscles will consume this glucose while you make kettlebell swings. This reduces the requirement for your body with diabetes to manage it, something it can't do by itself.

Benefit 8: Kettlebell training increases stamina for women.

Certain benefits that we've already discussed can contribute to the benefit of endurance. Kettlebell Swings aid in building more stamina in your body due to additional benefits that are associated with them, including an increase in muscle strength fitness, cardiovascular exercises, and an increase in lung capacity.

At first, you'll need those muscles that are strong, they will perform better. The more powerful your muscles are when kettlebell rotation, the more physical strength you will be able to produce. You'll be able to lift more weight or jump more, leap higher, and run faster thanks to kettlebell-swinging muscles.

Your muscles also require oxygen for their function, and that's where your robust heart and powerful lungs are at work. A lungs that is efficient when taught by kettlebells will absorb, process and transfer more oxygen into the body. The muscles require oxygen to prevent them from being tired. They can also stop the buildup of lactic acid which causes your muscles to burn.

In the end, the robust cardiovascular system that you get from the Kettlebell Swing gives you is essential to pump oxygenated blood to your muscles. As you can observe, the three of them can be described as stronger muscles, healthier heart and lungs that are stronger and all the advantages of kettlebell swings. All of which improve your capacity to exercise vigorously over time.

Benefit 9: Improve Your Ability to Balance

Another benefit of kettlebell swings is that they aid in improving your balance. When you perform the kettlebell swing, you're moving the kettlebell between your legs, while you're bent and holding the kettlebell above and ahead of your head. You do this with your arms extended and stretched out.

This constant and fast shifting of positions means your body must adapt to these shifts in position and move in a way that absorbs the shift in position and, consequently, your balance will be improved. Proprioceptors are the nerves in your muscles which are able to detect changes in position and are the mechanisms that make your body adapt to maintain its balance.

As you work your muscles or improve your memory The more you practice things that push you to be balanced and balance, the more stable your balance will get with time. Naturally, a strong balance is essential to a variety of aspects of your life. In addition, Kettlebell swings can help enhance your posture through strengthening of your back and core muscles. A strong core can pharmaceuticals to better posture and aids in keeping your balance in good shape.

Benefit 10: Weight Loss Goals

Another benefit to Kettlebell Swings is that they could help you shed a significant amount of weight. Simply simply put, your body requires the energy it needs to perform, and that energy is derived from the food you eat or, if there's an insufficient amount of calories within your body, it's by storing fat. In fact, the kettlebell exercise can produce up to 20 calories per minute. which means 300 calories over 30 mins, or 1,200 calories within an hour.

You may not want to go through a series of swings in 30 minutes but, if do, you'll reap huge benefits from burning calories. If you do not have enough calories in your body the body will use body fat to gain the energy it requires and remove the unwanted pounds that are accumulating that are weighing you down.

This Kettlebell Swing also helps to boost your metabolic rate as well as your EPOC. This means that your body burns more calories after your training is over as it would normally. The end result is that the Kettlebell is a great weight loss instrument. It is true that muscles burn fat, and when you build up with kettlebell exercises, the more fat you'll burn. That's an additional benefit.

Advantage No. 11: Reduction In Back Pain

The swinging motion that the kettlebell's rotation, when combined by the weight on the kettlebell can assist in reducing back pain that is caused by tight muscles and the dorsal load of discs. In short, this workout will help you extend your back muscles, loosen him and help him get back to normal.

The kettlebell swing is great exercise that has numerous advantages. The entire human body, from bottom to top will be benefited by the exercise. The benefits of Kettlebell Sings are certain to bring you happiness and better health!

Females are strong, and are able to lift more weights. One of the most commonly held beliefs about women is to only use tiny weights of 3 pounds to prevent mass formation. Like we said earlier women are not able to produce much growth hormone, therefore replenishment isn't a problem.

If you do kettlebell exercises correctly that is, you work your entire body, and you use your legs and hips and you burn lots of calories and employ a multitude of muscles simultaneously. You must lift higher weights in order to stimulate all of these muscles.

Here are the kettlebells that a females can utilize:

*8kg/15lbs - the take-off weight

*12kg/25lbs - Women who are athletic will reach this weight in just six weeks, particularly when swinging with two hands.

*16kg/35lbs for stronger women will utilize this weight to perform a number of exercises in the first 6 months of their lives.

The 7 best Kettlebell exercises To Do For Women

Below are the kettlebell workouts that help women the most. The order is priority, therefore begin then work your way through the list.

*KETTLEBELL SINGLE-ARM DEADLIFT

Muscles utilized: buttocks quads, thighs core, back

What is important: This is the single exercise that women of all ages should be focusing on is deadlifts. Deadlifting with just one arm is a great way to attention straight towards that back part of the body, and then into the glutes. If you want a powerful, elevated and stunning back it is what you need to perform.

One-arm deadlifts can also boost you heartbeat and also burn a lot of calories. Don't be afraid to add weight when you are able to master the method.

A KETTLEBELL LEG SINGLE DEADLIFT

Muscles to be used: glutes hips, thighs and back and core (front as well as back)

What is important The body connects hips and legs to the arms and shoulders through those muscles in the trunk. One-leg deadlifts work hard in the trunk muscles, connecting shoulders to hip opposite through the cross-body loop system.

The one-leg deadlift can not only create amazing torsos, but can also safeguard your spine from further training injuries. It's also an excellent exercise to strengthen the hips, buttocks and the hamstrings!

*KETTLEBELL SWING

Muscles that are used: Glutes Thighs The hips, quads, Core Back

What's important: After you've completed the two exercises listed above and you're ready to have fun, it's time to start. Kettlebell Swings quickly will become your primary exercise to burn fat.

Kettlebell Swings do not only help challenge over 600 muscles of the body but also provide cardiovascular benefits. Prepare yourself for strength, cardio and an extremely enjoyable workout all in one.

*KETTLEBELL TURKISH getting up

Muscles to be used: buttocks quads, hips, thighs core, triceps

Why is it important What is the significance of it? Turkish The Get Up a fantastic workout that goes deeply into the core muscles as well as improves flexibility of joints. If you've ever felt tight or slack, moving up can certainly assist.

The GetUp is an amazing exercise and can be enjoyed completed from start to finish. Spend time on the GetUp the body and mind will appreciate for it.

*KETTLEBELL SERIES

Muscles to be used: buttocks hips, thighs, quads, core back, shoulders, biceps, and shoulders.

What is the significance of it Why it is important: The series is a vital exercise that targets both the back and back shoulder. The sequence of exercises as illustrated below is also beneficial for the legs as well as the core.

The Row exercise can help you reduce your shoulders and enhance the appearance of your chest. It's also great for countering the sedentary lifestyle that many of us do each day.

*KETTLEBELL SQUAT and Press (BOW THRUSTER)

Muscles to be used: buttocks hips, thighs, quads core, triceps

What is the significance? There aren't many muscles free of the effects caused by Squat and Press. It is possible to do the exercise using one hand, then switch to the other after a set number of times or with two hands.

One of the biggest errors in this exercise is to not be sufficient depth to do squats. Do your best to lower your thighs until you reach the floor to get an additional glute-activation bonus.

*KETTLEBELL LATERAL LUNGE

Muscles employed: buttocks hips, thighs quads, core

What is important: The side-to-side failure does not just open your hips but also your large legs as well as a back that is raised. The more you can push the side tilt the better, but you must start slowly and gradually work your way more and more into the exercise each time.

*BONUS BONUS: A PUSH-UP

Muscles Used: Buttocks, Core, Chest, Triceps

The reason it is important: Men naturally have more muscular torso than women which is why they are more likely to avoid the from the pull-up. If you're looking to strengthen your core, chest and the back of your arms, then pushing-ups are crucial.

If you're struggling with pushups that are full, raise the hands to the table. When you are able to do 10 reps then lower your hands down to a bench, and then lower them to the ground.

Chapter 5: The Essentials Techniques

I thought it would be beneficial to go over a few fundamentals in regards in lifting heavy weights. If you're comfortable with the basics that you know, then skim this part, but skim it through quickly if you require an update.

These are the fundamental actions you must take when performing kettlebell training. These tips will help you keep yourself from injury and make the most from your workouts.

TUT is crucial for the growth of muscles TUT is essential for muscle growth. (TUT) is a common mistake I'm seeing often. A lot of beginners are unaware of the significance of TUT, and wonder why their results don't go as planned. Time under tension is exactly what it says the length of time that your muscles are under tension during an exercise. The longer the time of tension you can manage, the more you'll stimulate your the growth of your muscles.

I think that many people who are new to bodybuilding see professional bodybuilders exercising and doing their reps extremely quick. However, I believe they are missing the point professional bodybuilders who take steroids and perform fast reps as their gains are artificially aided. For the majority of us, slow repetitions will provide the greatest value for your money.

Most of often, based on the various exercises you'll be doing however, for the majority of the time , I suggest that you take 5 seconds to complete every movement you make with the weight. For instance, if you're doing the squat, lower your body for 5 seconds and then lift for five seconds.

There's an excellent article available from SimplyShredded.com which goes into more details about TUT in the section on resources.

Make sure you breathe properly - One of everything I would suggest that you breathe properly. If you're not breathing properly or aren't breathing properly while you exercise it will cause serious harm to your body in one way or the other. It's easy to be pulled by something if you're taking your breath in as you do exercises using the weight of a heavy object. This is the reason you should take your breath in and breathe in a manner that is safe to avoid serious problems in the future.

To properly breathe, you have to do two basic things. To make it easier to understand I will take the squat exercise that I previously used. As you lower your body as you perform the squat, you should breathe into. If you are bringing your body to the surface, we need to let out our breath. The same principle applies to any exercise, the example of doing the bench press. When you lower the weight, you breathe in, and as you push the weight upwards then you need to exhale.

Medium Grip - This is crucial when kettlebells. Depending on the kind of workout that you're performing, you'll typically need an average grip when holding the kettlebell. You should ensure that you're not gripping the kettlebell too tightly that you're holding it with a death grip however, you don't want to hold the kettlebell so loose that it will fall off your hands.

When you master some exercises, such as the kettlebell snatch, you'll understand why this is essential to understand. In general, some exercises require shifting your grip on the kettlebell in order to complete the exercise. Remember to most times keep your grip on the middle.

Keep your eyes up at the front of you. This point as well as the following point are the most important things to be doing to avoid injury when you work out. It is recommended maintain your straight head and your eyes focusing on the ahead of you, though certain kettlebell exercises require that you look at the kettlebell when you are doing the exercise. For the most part, you should keep your head straight especially when doing an exercise in which you're standing or bent over. This can help prevent injury in your neck or upper body.

Keep Your Back Straight Another thing to consider in order to avoid injuries during exercise is to stay back straight. This is recommended for virtually any exercise that you're performing. Imagine a line that is drawn across your back while you exercise. If you don't adhere to this, you could suffer from painful injuries that you might not be able to repair in the near future. It's easy to pull muscles if you do not follow this advice.

Chapter 6: Minor Body Kettlebell Exercises

Jerk Press (Shoulders)

Begin by using the handle of the kettlebell using one hand. Get rid of, i.e., lift the kettlebell by lifting it to the shoulder of your hand as you extend your legs and hips. Make sure to move your wrist around as you are doing this, i.e., the hand should end up facing the front of your body. This is your starting position.

If you keep your upper body straight then dip your body bend your knees.

Then, swiftly shift direction by pushing your heels into the ground to generate momentum. While doing this, lift the kettlebell in front of you by extensing your arm until it locks out. Make use of the force of your body to accomplish this.

When you return to the ground, take the weight immediately by getting into a squatting position under the kettlebell when your feet touch the ground. The idea of landing on your forefoot or the soles of your feet, not your heel - and then immediately letting yourself go into a squatting posture will reduce the risk of injuries to your knees and feet through an optimal shock absorption.

Return to a standing posture, Then lower the kettlebell towards your shoulder. This is the end of one repetition.

Perform between 8 and 10 repetitions for each shoulder or arm per set.

Jackknife Pull Over (Abdominals)

Begin by lying on your back and lie on the floor. Spread your legs completely, by putting both heels in contact with each with each other. Utilize both hands to hold the bulk of the kettlebell. Then, fully extend your arms to the side of your head. The kettlebell should have been in an even line between your body and your hands by the time you finish.

Start the exercise with "crunching" upwards, i.e., lifting up one leg and then both fingers off of the ground at once toward one another. At the top of the move, you will have your shoulder blades off of the floor, and your knees and hands close to one another. While you are performing this exercise be sure to exhale.

Gradually return to the beginning position and inhale whilst doing so.

Repeat the exercise by lifting the leg on the opposite side. It's a single repetition. Perform between 8 and 10 repetitions for each set.

One Arm Secure Chest Press (Chest)

Lay on your back on a flat bench or an mat for exercise.

If you hold a kettlebell, use one hand. Place your hand on the point of your nipple. Keep your arm with a 90-degree bent.

In addition to keeping your body steady with your legs and free arm and legs, pull the kettlebell upwards until your elbows come to a stop of locking out.

• Lower the kettlebell down back to its starting position slowly which is 1 repetition. Do 8 to 10 repetitions per arm for each set.

One-Arm Closed Row (Back)

Place a kettlebell behind your feet.

You can bend your knees a bit and then extend the butt to as far as you are able to be able to bend and then assume the position you started from. Maintain your spine straight all the time to reduce the risk of injury it.

In one hand, hold the kettlebell, and then move it towards your stomach and as you dothis, push the elbow back as far as you can and then lower your shoulder blade. Again, always keep your lower back straight.

- Lower the kettlebell without letting it go. Repeat. Perform 8 to 10 repetitions per arm for each set.

Chapter 7: Irritable Training

In addition to using kettlebells in your CrossFit programme, you can also utilize it when practicing and preparing for a different sport. CrossFit is frequently utilized by professionals who rely on their fitness levels to perform their job effectively. Policemen, firemen and paramedics take advantage of this program across the country. You'll benefit more through this exercise if participate in the sports the CrossFit community in your area plays.

If you include cross-training in your exercise routine You will expose your body different movements that challenge all of it. A focus on just a few muscles all the time is not enough for achieving general fitness. Many people feel out of fit when they try an exercise routine that is new or new exercise. Fitness enthusiasts who are familiar with working on his upper body might find themselves feeling really out of shape while jogging. If you place the bodybuilder into a game of running, such as basketball, they may feel unprepared due to the lack of training. They're not used to the speed or the agility required for the sport.

Cross-training can benefit. Through constant research of new workout routines and sports to test we can improve every aspect that make up our physical fitness. We also are increasing our capabilities not only on the sports field, but also with the physical demands of everyday life.

How do I start cross-training?

Training for two kinds of sports

You can pick the exercises suggested in this book to prepare for a particular sport. When you are studying a new sport make note of the fundamental movements you will need to master as well as the muscles you'll have to build in order to perform the movements with ease. Then, you should choose kettlebell exercises for the day that will focus on the movements you need to master.

Include speed and flexibility in your training

If you are doing cross-training it is important to not forget the other components of fitness that many muscle-builders do not consider: flexibility and speed. It is good to know that the exercises which improve these elements of fitness can be accomplished without the need for equipment.

Find a new sport to play every year

Most people are focused on three or four kinds of sports or exercises when they doing cross training. Many of them, however, are tired of these activities. The monotony of training contributes to the stiffness of joints, which reduces the flexibility and agility. For keeping your body in good shape and keep it challenging to the max, you must learn each year a new activity. Many people who have mastery of swimming in a sport, for instance and then go on to learn diving or surfing. Pick sports that are closely related to the sport you're pursuing.

Chapter 8: 13 Soviet Kettlebell Moves

Kettlebell Exercise No.1: Kettle Halo

The kettlebell halo is also called "around the globe" is a fantastic exercise to build core strength and strength in the shoulders. Take the kettlebell from the side of the horns and raise it up to chin-level in order to be standing it up on its side in a squat like a goblet. The kettlebell's bottom should be in the direction of the ceiling. The elbows need to be put with the rack in place. Move the elbows the other side and the kettlebell goes over your shoulder and back towards the back of the head. Keep your glutes tight and your abs strong. Also, be sure to keep your back straight. Lift the kettlebell to the other shoulder, then return to an upside-down goblet posture at the front of your body.

Then change direction and continue to move around your head, then back towards your chest. Your starting point is having both elbows in a tucked position at the chest. When you move, you release one, and then the other to allow for rotation. The path of the exercise as having a halo on top of your head. Make sure to keep the kettlebell near to your head during the exercise. Do not let your head shift during the exercise. focus on it straight ahead. It is helpful to choose an area on the wall directly in the front of you, and to keep your attention on it during the exercise. If you are required to look downwards and then lower the head, the kettlebell isn't heavy enough. Reduce the weight to enable the correct method of use.

Kettlebell Exercise No.2: Kettlebell Deadlift

The deadlift is an essential exercise to build muscles in the posterior chain which includes muscle groups of glutes, lower back and the hamstrings. The kettlebell variant also enhances the hip-expanding technique, which allows to perform better on exercises as cleans, snatches and swings.

Put this kettlebell between your legs, and close to your body. While your feet are shoulder-width apart, slouch back and relax your hips and allow yourself to slide down until you grasp the handle. Maintain your chest in a straight line throughout the entire movement. Grab the handle with both hands, and then get back to your standing position by putting your heels on the ground. The strength for lifting is derived from your glutes which must be squeezed tightly, as well as the lower part of your back (erector spine).

Then you will repeat the descent, pulling the hips forward and then slowly dropping until the kettlebell hits the ground. It is essential to keep your center of gravity in line with your body during this move. Additionally, you must be bending your body towards the hips instead of being bent at the waist. The lower back must be arched slightly throughout the entire movement. To focus on the hamstrings better ensure that your legs are straight throughout the entire movement. To put more focus on the glutesand hamstrings, lean your legs a bit when you descend. Keep your elbows straight and keep your keep your chest elevated throughout the exercise.

An alternative to this move is to do a double kettlebell deadlift. It involves by putting the kettlebells into the form of a bag that is lifted like a grocery store.

Kettlebell Exercise No.3: Two Handed Kettlebell Swing

The swing of the kettlebell is a traditional kettlebell exercise that can be used to build power. To master the technique, follow the steps in the following:

First step: With your your feet separated by a shoulder, put the kettlebell in between your feet. Like a deadlift, push your hips backwards to return towards the kettlebell (imagine that you're trying to shut the door of a car with the butt). Keep your head straight and ensure that your shoulders aren't above your knees. Take the kettlebell in an overhand grip that is two-handed. Lift yourself up to an upright position by flexing your hips while coming up. Repeat this five times, in rapid in rapid.

Step Two: Set the kettlebell further back so you have the handle aligned to your heels. Repeat the motion you've just done. You'll notice that, this time, you will notice an equilateral pendulum effect that is visible during the peak of your exercise. Then, try driving the kettlebell between your legs while going down to the point that it falls down underneath your butt. As you ascend, push the weight until it is the level of your shoulders. Make sure that you're not lifting using your shoulders or arms as the strength must come from your hips. This is one of the exercises where the swing of a pendulum is desirable. The use of momentum this way eases the stress to the upper back as well as grip as well as giving you more performance.

Kettlebell Exercise No.4: One Arm Straight and Clean

The one-arm clean is a fantastic intermediate movement between swing as well as pressing workouts. Once you are proficient in this exercise, you'll learn to create a rhythmic motion that moves from one rep to the next.

It is essential to maintain your grip loose on the kettlebell throughout the exercise. This will stop the kettlebell from hitting your forearm while you do the exercise. Begin by taking a slightly wider that shoulder-width stance with the kettlebell resting in between the legs. Then, with your hips tucked back, with your lower back slightly arched in order to lower your back and hold the kettlebell with an overhand grip and your thumb pointing behind you. The hand that is not working should be to your side, and your grip shut. Maintain a healthy back position by lifting your head.

Inhale while you scrub the kettlebell down to shoulder height. When you are rising the kettlebell should rotate in your hand to an unlocked position. When you lock out in the top the quads, glutes and hamstrings should be in good shape. As you ascend the kettlebell, it should be moving in a vertical direction up your body. In the highest position you should allow the kettlebell to rest on your forearm and chest in what is called the rack position. The kettlebell must now be placed in the triangle which is created by your chest, forearm and elbow.

One of the most frequent issues associated with this type of movement is the uncomfortable hitting the kettlebell with the forearm. It is because you are gripping the handle too tightly. Release the grip and allow your fingers to sink as deep as you can as the kettlebell gets up to chest height.

Kettlebell Exercise No.5: Single Press

Begin by placing the kettlebell in the upper spot of One Arm Clean (the rack position). You should have your elbow placed into your stomach. Your arms and wrists should remain straight. Place your arm that is not working towards the side for stability. Bring the kettlebell upwards in straight lines to ensure that your elbow remains locked in the top position. The hand should be set in a way that your thumb points at the opposite direction to your back. Make sure you're pushing your entire body instead of just your shoulders. The motion should include an exaggeration of lats as well as the extension and compression of the spine.

Reduce the kettlebell using moving your body backwards so that the kettlebell can return to its original position. The movement of lifting and lowering must be smooth and without movement that is jerks.

Breathing should follow a 4-stage pattern that follows:

(1) Breathe in deep while keeping the kettlebell in the rack position.

(2) Breathe out just before the overhead push.

(3) Inhale while you speed up

(4) Inhale as you secure your body from the top position

Kettlebell Exercise No.6: Snatch

The kettlebell snatch is based on the swing of the kettlebell Make sure your form is in line to swing prior into this exercise. With your feet about shoulder-width apart and the kettlebell in behind your heels. Then, you can push your hips back and lower the kettlebell. Keep your head elevated making sure that your shoulders don't go in the way of knees. Take the kettlebell in the one hand grip. Get yourself into an upright position swiftly by flexing your hips as you rise up. Be sure to keep your shins in a straight line throughout the move.

Find a great pendulum movement moving with a variety of swings, with your hips directing the motion, and the arms just steering. All should be locked in the highest position. After five or so swings you can take the kettlebell up until it's locked over your head. When you are up the kettlebell will move across your hand until, when in the lockout position, it's sitting on the upper arm's back. The top position of your hand should remain fully open. Re-grip as you go down. If you're doing high reps, you should hold the highest position for a moment or two in order to let your breath out. Alternate arms after every five overhead snatches.

Kettlebell Exercise No.7: Goblet Squat

It is the Kettlebell Goblet Squat is a great exercise for opening the hips and building power in the lower part of the body. With a slightly bigger than shoulder width grip, grasp the kettlebell with the horns, and keep the kettlebell at chest height. Maintain your elbows while you drop into the lunge. Engage yourself in pulling yourself down by using your glutes and your hips, moving out and back. Do not go too far back but you're looking to stay as straight as possible. Start straight downwards into an extended squat. The elbows should drop and rest in your knees, and on your thighs inside the lower squat position. This will stop the knees from collapsing. Your knees will move slightly forward, but they shouldn't go into the back. Bring your chest up and then look upwards from this position. In reality, they should be tracking your toes all the time.

When you are in the bottom position, move your knees side-to-side and use your elbows to push your joints apart. Pull your tailbone downwards and your head upwards.

Take your breath deeply, exhale, and then drive straight to the beginning position.

Kettlebell Exercise No.8 Windmill

The Windmill is an extremely efficient exercise to strengthen the glutes, hamstrings as well as the lower back and shoulders. It is also a great exercise for the core, in addition to making you more solid and steady when you are in an overhead position. This can also be a great method to improve your flexibility.

Begin in the rack position , with your feet shoulder-width apart. The kettlebell should be powered up until an overhead position locked out. Your feet should be at 45 degrees towards the arm that is in the position of holding your kettlebell. Transfer around 90% of your body weight onto the leg on the inside that will bear the weight. Then, kick the kettlebell's side hips out, and you lower to bring your non-kettlebell arm towards your toe, on the opposite side. Make sure the overhead arm is locked in as you lower. Be sure to look up throughout the move and use your legs as a guide to follow your arm towards your toe.

It's your choice whether you lock out your front leg. But the back leg should remain locked out during the entire motion. Don't shift your weight of on the front leg in the down portion of the motion. Instead, keep the focus on your rear foot by pushing the hips of the rear forward and up. Your shoulder will move when you push out your hip. Then bring your body back until the toe.

Kettlebell Exercise No.9: High Pull

It is the Kettlebell High Pull is a entire body workout that builds endurance and strength that makes you more agile for sports such like basketball, sprinting Karate and boxing.

When your feet are shoulder-width apart, put this kettlebell on your feet. Then, you can push your hips back and drop down to the kettlebell. Keep your head straight and ensure that your shoulders don't go over your knees. Take the kettlebell in two hands overhand grip near the top of the horns , so that your thumbs are in contact. Be sure that your shoulders are directly in front and behind the kettlebell. Start the pull by pushing downwards through your feet, and then pushing your hips up and towards the front. Your arms should remain extended throughout the initial portion of your pull. Utilize the power of the leg drive to raise your body. The kettlebell should be lifted to the level of your chest. Then let your momentum lift you to your feet, and then lower yourself to your starting position. While in the top place, you elbows must be lifted above your weight.

Kettlebell Exercise No.10: Turkish Get Up

It is said that the Turkish Get Up can be a fantastic full body workout. It is excellent to build cardiovascular endurance as well to build functional strength and strength.

Begin by lying down on the ground, lying on your back, with your knees bent. The kettlebell should be lying on the floor on your right. Put your right hand completely into the handle of the kettlebell, and bring the weight up to your chest. With both shoulders on the floor, lift your left arm upwards to ensure that the kettlebell is directly over your chest. Your the right leg should bend in such a way that your right foot is lying flat on the floor. Your left hand should lie sitting flat on the ground at a 45 degree angle.

From the beginning place, you should rise onto your left elbow while making sure that your right arm is fixed. Then, rise to the point that you can support your body only with your left hand and right foot. The left foot should remain straight, and just a few inches above the floor. Move your butt and leg backwards to place your knee to the left on floor. Now you can rise to a lunge position using your left hand to get off the floor , and the contact points are both your left foot and the left shin.

The kettlebell remains in the overhead position.

Then, by pushing off the back leg lift yourself to standing. Focus on the kettlebell all the time. Reverse the movement to return to your beginning position.

Kettlebell Exercise No.11: Russian Twist

It is believed that the Russian Twist is a very excellent exercise for building core strengthwhile also making the obliques more defined and shape. Stand up straight on the floor, with kettlebells beside you as you tilt your back slightly to ensure your abs are stretched to keep you moving. Bend your knees while by keeping your legs together, raise your feet about six inches above the ground. Take hold of the kettlebell using an overhand grip toward one of the upper horns. Beginning with the kettlebell seated on your waist, move it towards the right side to lower the weight until it reaches the floor. If it touches the floor, move to the opposite side, and then touch the floor there.

Repeat this process while making sure to bring the kettlebell down to the floor every time. It is important to ensure that your feet remain off the ground during the entire exercise.

Kettlebell Exercise No.12: Two Arm Kettlebell Row

This is an excellent exercise to build strength and functional strength of the muscles of the upper shoulders, back and arms. Begin by placing a pair kettlebells on the ground wide enough to walk through them. While keeping your heels on the ground then bend your knees to grasp the handles of the kettlebells. Your hips should track back, and keep the arch of your back as you lower. After that, soften your knees and lift your glutes up. This will create a flat back posture. Then breathe as you bring the arms toward your chest. Make sure to keep the tension in your muscles of the back and in that of upper-arm muscles. Keep the kettlebells in check when you return them to their starting position. Do not let your shoulders move forward.

Kettlebell Exercise No.13: Lunge Clean / Lunge Press

This is a fluid move that gives you the chance to do the best cardio and power combination exercise. It's great for the lungs and heart as well as is an excellent fat-burner. Start by putting an exercise kettlebell to your right hand, with the feet spaced shoulder-width apart. Begin to lunge forward with your left leg. After you have completed the lunge, remove the kettlebell from the right side of your shoulder. Continue to move forward by lunging using the left leg. Once you have completed this lunge, lift the kettlebell upwards. Continue this lunge-clean-lunge-process for the required time allotment.

Chapter 9: Huge Muscles And Kettlebells

What exactly are Big Muscles?

Muscles are generally split into small and large muscles. Big muscles consist of quadriceps, glutes, chest, back and the hamstrings. On the other hand small muscles are comprised of triceps and shoulders and biceps. They also include calves. To train it is essential to examine how different muscle groups can perform in the course of exercise and then select the muscles being working the most. However, it is advised to select large muscles in order for greater intensity during workout. The reason behind this is that larger muscles enable the body to be active without the body being exhausted because of smaller muscle activity. It also allows the individual to lift more weight and to control their body. In turn, it increases the capacity to coordinate movements and decrease the risk of injuries. While small muscles serve to support for larger muscles during training and are unable to work at high intensity. Because of this, the growth of small muscles is restricted.

Furthermore, there are many methods to maximize the benefits by separating the training for the larger and less muscle groups during different times. This will make sure that each muscle is being trained to maximum capacity. If this isn't an alternative, then one can split training into courses of 4 weeks in which there is one week to small muscle training, and three weeks for large muscle training. The principal reason for using these muscles is because they help to burn fat and increases the strength. Since muscles are utilized in the exercise routine, it helps to build muscle mass and the muscle tissue results in burning more calories.

To burn off fat, it is essential to include exercise for strength and cardio since it makes use of large muscles and can help improve performance. For instance having strong glutes to go running can help you run faster over a longer time and burns off more calories. Likewise, performing exercises that strengthen your core will help keep your fitness for biking. This helps you burn more calories.

How Kettlebell helps to burn fat

The kettlebell is a reliable device that is able to strengthen the large muscles group. Kettlebells are regarded as the most efficient method which can assist in burning fat in the body, while not losing mass or muscle mass. It also allows for an athletic motion as well as improve low-back stability. It is due to the fact that swings are strong and involves large muscles and smaller muscles that helps to strengthen the muscles. Additionally, due to its athletic and dynamic movement, it lets the body produce the desired outcome based on the type of body. It also connects the upper part of the body with the lower body and creates functional strength rather than combining different body components.

Additionally the kettlebell swing also helps to burn calories within a short period of time as well as create muscles mass. It also assists in creating high heart rates using the use of relative light weights. The swing also improves the body while also improving cardiovascular strength and endurance. Numerous studies have shown that 20 minutes of kettlebell exercise could produce the same amount of calories as running at a 6-minute mile pace. But the speed that an individual is able to burn fat is a challenge to to determine, but when the exercise is of a high intensity and a strict diet is maintained, you can expect to lose approximately 1 to 2 pounds each week. While kettlebells typically produce more results, the time to burn fat is different because of the variety of elements involved in kettlebell workout.

Chapter 10: Mistakes To Circumvent

Individuals who are brand new to exercising must take the time to master the proper technique and avoid errors. It is very easy to suffer injuries if you're doing exercises wrongly.

Incorrect movement pattern

Some people may be enticed to attempt exercises that are not suitable for their fitness levels. It is possible to cause back injuries. For instance, beginner should learn to master dead lifts prior to the swing.

What to do to prevent:

Beware of this error by learning slow. You can view videos to learn how to move.

Not maintaining neutral spine

In keeping your neck neutral position ensures you are in the correct alignment. It is important to keep this in mind when performing kettlebell exercises for intermediate levels like high pulls, swings and clean. If your body isn't correctly aligned, the entire spine as well as the muscles surrounding it could suffer injuries.

What to do to stay clear of:

Be sure to keep your head and hips in straight lines. Maintain your spine straight.

A too wide stance

Most kettlebell exercise requires the feet to be away from each other. But, having a an stance that is not wide enough could lung to injuries. Risk areas include knees, hips and lower back.

What to do to avoid:

Be sure to maintain an athletic posture. It's when your legs are separated and will make it simple to jump.

Squeezing the bell using the upper part of your body

Be careful not to over emphasize the muscles in your upper body as this can affect the efficiency of your workout and could put strain on your body. It is possible to suffer shoulder, neck and lower back injuries when you put too much emphasis upon your upper part of the body.

What to do to prevent:

Be sure to relax your upper back and make sure to lock your knees out for each repetition.

Training until muscles fail

It is crucial to push yourself every time you do a set, however you shouldn't experience any extreme pain while exercising. If you exert yourself too hard you are more prone to injury and fatigue of muscles.

What to do to prevent:

Rest after a few repetitions.

The attempt to salvage a bad repetition

Be aware of your movements. If something doesn't feel correct, stop and look at your posture or the way you hold the kettlebell prior to returning to the workout.

What to do to avoid:

Don't try to force poor repetitions. Always keep an eye on your posture while working out.

Try anything extravagant

Making up fancy movements which are not the standard movements in exercising can be extremely risky. Your body may not be ready to perform the workout and could cause a spinal injuries. There are many things that can be wrong when you attempt to perform impromptu and bizarre moves with kettlebells.

What to do to prevent:

Make sure to stick to the fundamental movements in the most extent you can since they work most efficiently. Include the fundamental principles of kettlebell exercises even when you attempt more challenging movements.

With a firm grip

If you grip the handle too tightly, it is ineffective and risky. It is possible to sustain injuries to your elbow and hand.

What to do to prevent:

Take your hands off your shoulders and grip the handle using your fingers instead of your palms.

Smacking the forearms

A few kettlebell exercise routines such as cleaning and grasping change the direction of the bell throughout the exercise. The bell should be controlled so that it doesn't drop and hit your arms.

What to do to prevent:

Lift the kettlebell up instead of swinging it over the top. Relax your grip and let the kettlebell fall in your forearm.

Wearing improper footwear

Unfit footwear doesn't just include slippers or open toe sandals. Shoes for running are also not recommended for kettlebell exercises as they could raise the heel and push the knee up when squatting, which could lead in knee injuries.

What to do to avoid:

Make sure you train using flat soled sneakers.

Chapter 11: Types Of Kettlebells

There are a variety of kettlebells. The most well-known kinds are powder coat kettlebells and cast iron kettlebell and steel competition kettlebell.

Powder coat kettlebell

The main difference between a powder-coated kettlebell and a cast iron kettlebell is the coating of powder that helps to make it more sturdy. The color-coded bands on the handles signify the the weight.

Cast iron kettlebell

They are often employed to build muscle. They come with thick and smooth handles that are designed to avoid the chafing. They feature a flat bottom to make it easy to store. The kettlebells are weighed in kilograms and the sizes are based on their weight. The kettlebells used for exercise depends on the person and how much one wishes to push the shoulders.

Steel competition kettlebells

They're all of the same size regardless of weight. Therefore, every weight can be able to fit into your hands exactly the same way. Color codes match according to international standards.

Kettlebells coated in rubber, as the name implies come coated with rubber, and do not rust.they also aren't scratched. They are available in different sizes based on the weight.

The kettlebells made of vinyl are coated with vinyl, a synthetic resin that is made up of various colors that give an elegant look.

Classic kettlebells expand in size when the weight grows. A kettlebell of 50kg is more than a kettlebell that weighs 10kg.

Lifting Techniques

The following steps will guide you through the correct posture and how to perform the most common kettlebell exercises. If you're new to kettlebell exercises, it is advised to have a mentor or coach who is experienced with the exercises since the incorrect posture can pain to back pain.

This can happen when there is a lot of pressure put on the posterior chain during the swings. When using kettlebells, it is essential to have the correct technique and awareness of the proper posture, grip balance and the proper transitions. Similar to other exercises equipment, it is crucial to know how to properly utilize kettlebells in order in order to avoid injuries and guarantee a productive workout. There are excellent DVDs to assist in learning the correct techniques for handling kettlebells however one will need to consult an instructor who is certified to master the proper movements and safely perform them.

Style

There are three distinct styles of lifting kettlebells that have slightly different outcomes.

Hard-style. It is believed to be the first kettlebell workout that produces massive strength and explosive power. The Kime method is the underlying principle of hard style. It's an all-out effort for every repetition. The objective is to create the strength required for swinging, grasping press, or squat. However, the power increase is crucial. This type of training focuses on fast, rigid movements as opposed fluid and smooth movements. It is the reason it's also known as"the" Russian kettlebell competition. The hard styles increase both extremes of the strength and tension, while focused on speed and relaxation. The tighter the muscle is the greater the force generated. They boost strength by making contact with muscles more vigorously. Every workout results in greater output, but in shorter time.

The sports style. This style is a combination of strength and power to increase overall endurance. It requires the athlete to be able to carry a maximum load, and to lift the kettlebell in as many instances as they can within a time limit of 10 minutes.

Juggling. It's crazy to think of the concept of to juggle a steel ball weighting 10 or 20 pounds however it is the most popular form for kettlebell lifts. It improves the strength of the core and also the resistance of rotation. It also improves hand-eye coordination, and provides strong pulling strength, and most importantly, enjoyment.

HOLDS

The kettlebell can be used in a variety of ways to get various outcomes. What you do with it it, grip, grab and angle will determine the muscle to be employed and the amount of effort to be expected. The use of one hand or both hands during training can affect the results.

Racked. In this position you bend your arms, with the upper arm firmly held to the body, and the hand positioned in line to the neck. The handle is inside your palm, and the bell is placed on the outside.

Through the horns. This is a typical starting point and involves holding the kettlebell with the horns. The kettlebell is held close to the chest.

Crush or squeeze. It's like the way you hold a bell the horns. However, instead of gripping the horns, you grip the bell with your fingers by pressing it using the tips of your fingertips. This lack of grip makes it necessary for your arm muscles to adjust.

Waiter. The kettlebell was designed to fit in your palm.

POSTURE

While using kettlebells, it is essential to keep the correct posture in order to avoid injuries. The first consideration is to avoid hunching forward while wearing shoulders that are round. The head should be orientated toward the forward direction with the eyes focusing approximately 6 feet ahead. The spine should be in the normal S curve. This posture makes you appear as if you're waiting to get in the chair. If you're in that position, must be able to position a wooden stick on your spine from your neck towards your hips and make contact with your head shoulders and the upper glutes.

Chapter 12: Kettlebell Workouts For Newbie

The next chapter will be devoted to I'll aid you in starting I'll present you with three kettlebell exercises that anyone could perform.

Upper body

Core

Lower body

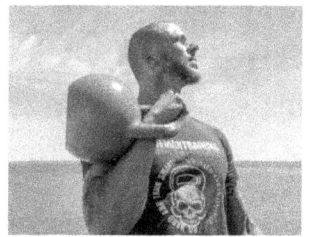

Beginners should begin easy and slowly. Before you bring the kettlebell in do the exercises without the weight added. Be aware of your body's movement through the movements, and be aware of any instability or balance issues. Improve your posture and make sure you're practicing correctly before doing any exercise with your kettlebells. Be sure to master your technique in order to avoid injury and to maximize the benefits of your kettlebell exercise.

TIP: It's beneficial to schedule a time of a few minutes with an instructor to help improve your technique. A professional will be able to observe your movements objectively from different angles and give direction to make sure you're doing each move within an exercise properly.

Squats and Lunges: When doing squats or lunges make sure to only do the exercise until it is comfortable. If you're experiencing problems with knee joints, make sure to keep your squats, lunges and squats higher to prevent discomfort. As you gain strength and stronger, you should try taking your squats lower if you are able. If you're unable to go any lower, you must perform these exercises on a pace that you feel comfortable with.

When to increase your weight or reps When to increase reps or weights: Refer chapter 8 to get guidelines for when you should increase the weight on your kettlebells or sets, repetitions and sets.

THE RACKED POSITION

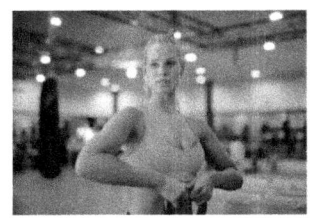

I will refer to the racked position in the following three chapters on kettlebell exercises. It is essential to learn the racked position and improve it. This way, you can prevent bruising and injury.

Hold the kettlebell's handle in such a way it is positioned on your palm diagonally. Your handle must pharmaceuticals through the crook of your thumb on one side , to the base of your palm and your wrist to the other.

In the racked hold position in which your kettlebell is positioned, it is placed against your chest at shoulder height , with the elbow bent. The kettlebell's body rests on your forearms' outer edges.

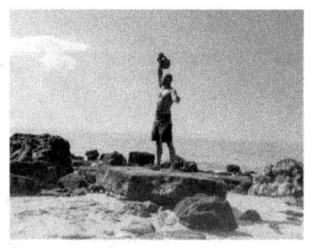

Form POOR RACK

If the racked hold isn't done properly, you could be injured because you put too much stress on your wrists elbow, forearm and shoulder. There are two main reasons to use an improper rack form.

The handle of your kettlebell is placed in the middle of your palm, not diagonally.

The kettlebell is being held towards the side, closer to your shoulder, but not close enough to your chest.

FLOPPING

If you are using the racked position in exercises, it's crucial to be aware of your grip on the handle while it turns in your palm. If you lower your kettlebell out of a Racked position the handle will move in your palm to push the kettlebell inwards. If you bring your kettlebell back up to the racked posture, the handle will naturally spin within your palm to turn the kettlebell to the rear the palm of your hands. It will then rest against your forearm's outside.

If you aren't able to exercise control of your grip, you may be prone to slapping the kettlebell on your outer forearm as you bring them into the rack grip. This can be a very painful experience and usually leaves bruises. However, the positive aspect is that when the strength of your grasp and grip over the kettlebell increase the likelihood is that you'll be able to stop the slide.

BEGINNER AUGMENTING BODY KETTLEBELL TRAINING

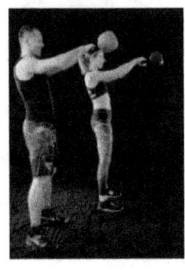

BEGINNER UPER BODY KETTLEBELL TRAINING

SETS FOR EXERCISE REPS

Pull Up 8-10 3 5

Press 8-10 per side, 3 5

Clean 8-10 per side, 3 to 5

Regular Row 8 - 10 for each side 3 5

Pull Over 8-10 3 5

The rest period between sets is 30 seconds to 2 minutes. Reduce your rest time as you progress and you get stronger.

PULLL UP

Muscles targeted: shoulders glutes, upper back quads, hamstrings

Holding the handle of your kettlebell tightly using both hands, stand with it hanging on top of your body. The kettlebell should hang around the thigh.

The kettlebell should be brought up to your chest, bent your elbows in a sideways manner. Once the kettlebell has reached the height of your chest and your arms are in line with the ground.

Move your arms upwards and lower your kettlebell until it is at thigh height.

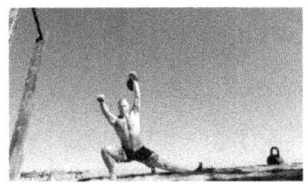

Alternate: Squat Pull Up

You can add some leg power to your pull up by doing an squat with your kettlebell that is suspended at thigh-height. When you are pushing into the squat, lift your kettlebell and pull it up position. When you lower your kettlebell to its thigh-height Squat down and repeat.

Press Release

Muscles to be targeted: shoulders core, triceps

Place your feet shoulder-width apart. Start by holding your kettlebell in a racked posture.

Move your arm to the side and raise your kettlebell up to the ceiling. Make sure to keep your kettlebell straight to your shoulders so that your elbow, shoulder and wrist are aligned with one another.

Bring your kettlebell down towards the Racked position.

Alternate: Push Press

To add some energy for your presses, you can perform an incline half squat, while holding the kettlebell in the rack posture. As you raise your body to the half-squat position position to standing, you can use the force to raise your arms into the press.

CLEAN

Muscles targeted: Shoulders back and core, quads glutes, hamstrings, and hamstrings.

Keep your feet shoulder width apart, keeping your kettlebell with the rack position. This is the exact position you'll complete the exercise in.

Move your elbow to the side and move your kettlebell into an upward angle. When it's swinging downwards make sure you bend your knees to move your torso forward with your hips, allowing the kettlebell to move through your legs.

When your kettlebell begins to swing forward then straighten your legs and bring your torso to a standing position. As you straighten up, push your hips upwards, the strength generated by the thrust of your hips can boost the momentum of the kettlebell's upward swing.

As the kettlebell swings upwards Bend your elbow and return it to the racked posture.

REGULAR ROW

Muscles to be targeted: shoulders core, biceps, back glutes, quads glutes, hamstrings

You should be in a comfortable, neutral position, with your feet shoulder-width apart, and place your kettlebell in between your feet.

Bend your knees, then pivot forward from your hips.

Grab your kettlebell using one hand.

The kettlebell should be pulled towards your ribs, bending your elbow while pulling it towards the ceiling.

Keep your elbow in place with your body to stop your arm going towards the side.

Lower the kettlebell by stretching your arm once more, but do not place your kettlebell to the ground. Keep it about 1 inch above the floor.

While doing the row exercise Maintain a straight back while keeping your shoulders at a level. Don't allow that arm's shoulder that you are lifting your kettlebell with to sink.

Alternate: Double Kettlebell Row

If you own two kettlebells with similar weight, you can complete the row with two kettlebells to enhance the difficulty of the exercise.

Pull OVER

Muscles to be targeted: shoulders the triceps muscles, back, core

Begin by lying in a position on your back, with your kettlebell placed on the floor, above your head.

Move your arms up above your head and grab your kettlebell , positioned on both sides of the handle.

Keep your arms straight and move your kettlebell upwards to your shoulders and then over the top of your head, until you have straight arms. Your elbows, wrists and shoulders must be in alignment with one the other.

The kettlebell should be lowered to the ground just above your head, but don't set it down. Keep the kettlebell about an inch above the floor.

Variation of Pull Over the hip Raise

As you advance, you can make your pull over do double duty. Once you've raised the kettlebell, you should hold the position. When you are in this position, you must keep your legs together, and lift the weight off the floor to make sure your legs are pointed upwards towards the ceiling. Engage your core muscles to lift your hips and legs above the flooring for a period in one, before dropping your hips , then straightening your legs to the floor.

BEGINNER CORE Workout

BEGINNER CORE Workout

SETS FOR EXERCISE REPS

Windmill 4 to 5 per side, 3 5

Lunge with a rotation of 8-10 3 5

Sit up from 8 to 10.3 - 5.

Carry of the farmer 45-60 seconds per side , 3 5

Figure eight 8 - 10 in each direction (left and right) 3 - 5

The rest period between sets is 30 seconds to 2 minutes. Reduce your rest time as you progress and you get stronger.

WINDMILL

Muscles to be targeted: shoulders, glutes, core and glutes, hamstrings

Place your feet shoulder width apart, your weight placed on your right hip, and your left leg is slightly extended towards the side.

Place your kettlebell on the rack position using the right side of your hand.

Reach your right arm out to lift your kettlebell over your head. Make sure to keep the kettlebell to your shoulders so that your elbow, shoulder and wrist are aligned with one another.

Arms on your left should be extended to your side.

Your torso should be rotated slightly to pull your left shoulder forward.

Turn your body to the left and then push your weight onto the right side of your hip.

Bend your knees as much as you feel comfortable. If you're not able to be able to touch the ground, that's fine.

Keep your right arm straight with your kettlebell hanging overhead. Do not bend your elbow or let your arm lean.

Straighten back up to the beginning position.

LUNGE WITH ROTOR

Muscles targeted: shoulders quads, core, glutes, hamstrings

Make sure your feet are wide apart.

Hold the kettlebell in both hands on the opposite end of the handle, and then hold it against your chest.

In a lunge position, you can do this by either returning to the reverse lunge or moving forward into a normal lunge.

While you do the lunge, move your torso so that you're looking out to the side but without moving your head.

Remain in a standing position and then rotate your body back towards the front while doing so.

Tips: If turning your torso as you perform the lunge becomes too hard Perform the lunge and hold it while rotating your body. Turn your torso towards the front, before returning to your starting position.

STAND UP

The muscles targeted are: core, back shoulders, back

Put your feet on the ground. Your legs must be straight ahead of you or bent at your knee, which is similar to the posture used for regular sit-ups.

Grab your kettlebell from the opposite hand and lower it to your chest.

Lay back on the floor, and then hold your kettlebell on your chest.

Perform a standard sit-up with your kettlebell held lightly on your chest. Do not push it towards the side or allow it to slide in your lap.

Then lower yourself back to the floor.

Make sure you engage your core muscles when performing the sit-up, avoid your lower back muscles to avoid injury.

FARMER'S CARRY

Targeted muscles: Core shoulder, obliques, forearms, shoulders

Place the feet spread shoulder width apart, and your kettlebell is securely held with one hand to your side.

Move forward and engage your core muscles in order to keep your body straight. Maintain your shoulders at a level. Avoid leaning to the side, or backward or in the direction of forward.

Make sure your kettlebell is as steady as you can during the entire time. It is possible to need to keep it a bit to your back in order to stop it from bouncing.

Instead of repeated sets Each set will comprise of walking around with the kettlebell for 45-60 minutes.

FIGURE-EIGHT

Muscles to be targeted: core, glutes, shoulders Quads and glutes, hamstrings

Keep the feet slightly larger than shoulder width apart with your knees bent slightly and the torso swayed forward from your hips.

Holding your kettlebell with your right hand, move it to your left from the front to the back.

While you move the kettlebell on towards your right side extend the right side of your hand through your legs and transfer your kettlebell in your left while it travels behind the left leg.

With your left hand, pull your kettlebell towards your legs. Then, turn it on the right hand side of your body from forward to back.

Place the left side of your hand through your legs in order to return it by transferring it from the right to your left while it swivels across the back of your right leg.

The kettlebell is carried in a figure-eight-like motion in between your legs.

Keep a straight back all the way through.

BEGINNER LOWER BODY Workout

BEGINNER LOWER BODY Workout

SETS FOR EXERCISE REPS

Two-handed Kettlebell Swing 8-10 3 5

Two-handed deadlift 8-10 3 - 5

Goblet squat 8-10 3 - 5

Two-handed lunge 8 - 10 3 - 5

Side Lunge 8 - 10 per side 3 - 5

Bob and weave 8-10 times to each side, 3 to 5

The rest period between sets is 30 seconds to 2 minutes. Reduce the time between sets as you progress and you get stronger.

TWO-HANDED SWING KETTLEBELL

Muscles to be targeted: quads glutes, hamstrings and shoulders Core and back

Place both feet about shoulder-width apart knees bent slightly and your torso swaying towards the front from your hips. Maintain your back straight as your torso hinges forward.

Hold the top of the kettlebell's handle using both hands.

Take your kettlebell off the floor and let it slide back and forth across your back.

Straighten yourself up to a standing posture and then thrust your hips inwards. The thrust of your hips will provide an energy boost to your kettlebell swing.

The kettlebell should be thrown out towards you with an arched motion until it is at the level of your chest, with your hands straight.

When your kettlebell begins to swing downwards once more you can bend your knees and move your torso forward by hinges by your hips. Then allow the kettlebell to move between your legs.

TWO-HANDED DEADLIFT

Muscles targeted: glutes, hamstrings, quads, back, core

You should be in a comfortable, neutral posture; feet shoulder width apart, and your kettlebell at your feet.

Bend your knees, and then hinge your torso inwards from the hips. Maintain your back straight.

Grab your kettlebell with firm grips on the handle using both hands.

Straighten yourself into a sitting position by lifting the kettlebell alongside your. The kettlebell should be hanging directly in front of you at a level that is thigh-high.

Bend your knees, and then hinge your torso inwards from your hips until you can place the kettlebell back between your feet.

GOBLET SQUAT

Muscles targeted: Hamstrings, glutes, quads, core

Place your feet at a distance of about shoulder width. Grab your kettlebell from the opposite handle's side and then place it upside-down against your chest.

Bend your knees and bring your torso inwards from the hips to complete the Squat.

Return to a standing posture.

Alternative: Goblet Squat Press

To make your goblet more interesting, add some spice to your squat, consider adding the press into your workout. If you are able to push yourself from the squat position to stand and raise your kettlebell above your head to press. Bring your kettlebell down to chest level prior to your next set of squats.

TWO-HANDED LUNGE

Muscles targeted: shoulders glutes, glutes, core and quads

Place your feet at a distance of shoulder width. Hold your kettlebell either side of the handle , and place it on your chest.

Move into a lunge posture by either returning to the reverse lunge or moving forward into a normal lunge.

Return to standing.

Variation: Double Kettlebell Lunge

If you own two kettlebells that are similar weight, you can keep both kettlebells by your sides during the lunge to provide additional resistance and challenge.

SIDE LUNGE

Muscles to be targeted: glutes quads, hamstrings, shoulders and back. Core,

Your feet should be at a distance of shoulder width. Hold your kettlebell either side of the handle , and keep it in your chest.

Move to your right, while benting your right knee before lower the body to a side lunge while keeping the left foot extended towards the side. Bring your hips back and pull your torso slightly to the side during the lunge.

Keep your kettlebell in a high position against your chest to avoid unnecessary stress on your lower back.

Return to standing.

Variation: Side Lunge Press

Increase your side lunge one notch. Keep the side lunge in place while lifting your kettlebell to the ceiling in order for presses. The kettlebell will be lowered to chest height prior to returning it back into a sitting posture.

BOB and WEAVE

Muscles targeted: hamstrings, glutes, quads, core, back

Place your feet shoulder-width apart, holding your kettlebell to either hand and placing it on your chest.

With your left leg, make a long step to the left.

As you walk, move your torso to the side from the hips and then 'duck' into an squat-like position, before straightening up and then bringing one leg forward side to take a stand.

While performing the bob and weave, imagine there's a low beam right next to you. You must get to the opposite part of the beam moving towards the side and then sliding under the beam then straightening yourself to the opposite face of the beam.

Chapter 13: Choosing Kettle Bells

Kettlebells are weights having the shape of a circle, made from cast iron and have a handle attached that allows users to get grips with ease. They have been in use for many years, but gained popularity just recently. The most popular and distinctive feature of this product is the ability to make use of active movements to build endurance, strength as well as agility and balance. Many are now using it due to its being powerful as well as challenging and practical. It can be held by either hand or both hands when performing various pulling, swings, and presses.

There are certain moves that call that the body weight be moved from one to another when you move the body up or the holder is moved in a lateral movement. This requires that the user maintains a steady body weight and exercises their abdominal muscles in an manner that is different from the normal.

Some movements require the strength or power that is derived from the hips as well as the lower extremities. This allows for the movement of the body's weight, providing it with coordinated bodily actions which are not usually included in other exercise routines.

The difference between dumbbells and kettlebells

A few people might think that kettlebells are a dumbbell of some sort however it's not. In certain ways they might be similar however, the kettlebell is distinct shape. It could appear to be an ordinary weight, however its unique shape affects how the weight is developed the body. Because the center of mass for kettlebells lies located outside of its hand, the weight is able to shift depending on the manner in which it is handled and moved. It's not the same for dumbbells, in which they have a center point that is in the hands or the hand of the individual using the kettlebell.

Kettlebell movements create an energy centrifugal force that is focused on stabilizing and decelerating muscles. This isn't the main idea in long-running strength-training programs. The kinds of exercises that use kettlebells involves a variety of directions that individuals are able to perform during their everyday life. For instance, someone carries a tiny suitcase to place within a container above the head. Another example is lifting overstuffed bags of luggage or grocery bags filled with a lot of things.

If kettlebells are regularly used they provide nearly the same advantages in terms of both functional and actual strength. The dumbbells help build muscles by using gentle and controlled exercises. However kettlebell exercises make use of all body parts and focuses on building strength as well as dynamic movements and endurance. The distinctive shape of the kettlebell permits to smoothly transition between exercises without the need to set the apparatus on the floor. This continuous technique, also known as "kettlebell flow" is believed to lead in greater metabolic burning and growth of more muscles in significantly less time.

Guidelines for selecting the appropriate weights

Kettlebells are available in various styles and weights starting from five pounds. They can be progressively heavier in increments of five pounds to more than 100 pounds. When choosing the right weight, ensure that it is sufficient in weight but not too strenuous for your exercise. The process of determining the correct weight could be a little difficult initially but, eventually you'll realize that each kettlebell exercise requires a certain amount of weight. For newbies, many of the ballistic exercises such as swing and push press might seem a bit awkward and unfamiliar and therefore, instructors advise beginning with light weights in order to learn the technique initially.

Guidelines for choosing your weight

5-10 lbs in women who have just beginning to train

10 to 15 pounds for women who are familiar with kettlebell exercises or for those who are new to kettlebells

20-25 lbs for women who have had previous experiences with kettlebells or for men with experience with kettlebells

30 lbs or more is for people who feel physically fit enough and have done kettlebell exercises in the past

For those who wish to take part in this type of training regularly it is necessary to use various weights that are suited to the kind of exercise to be completed. If you're not sure, begin by doing light weight exercises to become familiar with the movements prior to deciding to go with a more heavy weight. They can be found at a variety of sporting goods stores and online retailers. These may be costly, but they are a great option to train for strength exercises too.

Chapter 14: Burpees (Assemble Up To Doing This With 2 Kettlebells)

Fantastic way to finish off the last of a training session

A great alternative to boring cardio as you can get many things by doing burpees in short bursts.

Set a goal for 20 reps and 3 sets or intervals with timed timing (3x3mins.)

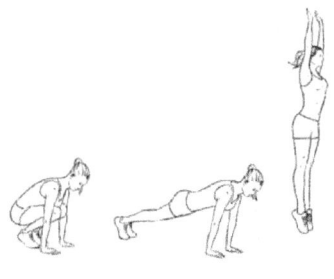

Straighten your legs, with your shoulders apart, and your hands at your sides.

In one easy motion, you will squat and then place your hands on the floor, right in the direction of your feet.

Move forward until your weight is in your hands. You should be at the same time , extending your legs behind you until they're fully extended. Your body should be in an unison line, with your weight resting on your toes as well as the soles of your feet as well as your arms extended. In essence, you should be in a push-up posture.

Jump your feet using your legs to spread to the point that they are more than the hip width, and then instantly jump them back to join them.

Complete one push-up in full.

Move your feet forward and place them just behind your hands.

Utilize a slam-dunk movement to press through your heels before returning to your starting point.

Repeat.

Exercise Toolkit

Alongside the previously detailed and illustrated three main movements from the kettlebell swing kettlebell Turkish getup, and kettlebell squat presse, below are some additional combinations of great compound movements that you can add to your arsenal. Each exercise is designed to activate the maximum amount of muscles in the most efficient, practical way.

Complex Moves to Target Your Back

Renegade Row

Excellent for stabilizing the core.

Fantastic compound move where you work multiple muscles in one move.

Balance is improved when you use two kettlebells.

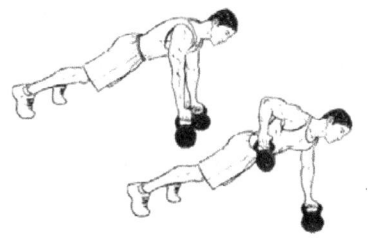

The addition of push-ups to the workout makes for fantastic back and chest exercises.

Set a goal of 20 reps, and 3 sets.

Two kettlebells should be placed on the ground, about an inch apart.

In a push up posture you should place your hands onto the grip portion of each Kettlebell to support yourself.

Set your legs just a little wider than the hip length apart, and your toes helping to support your weight. This is your starting point.

Pull down on one kettlebell while you simultaneously "row" the other kettlebell upwards by stretching your shoulder while bend your elbow.

The kettlebell should be lowered to the floor without stopping and repeat the exercise with the other hand.

If you've completed both arms, that's one repetition.

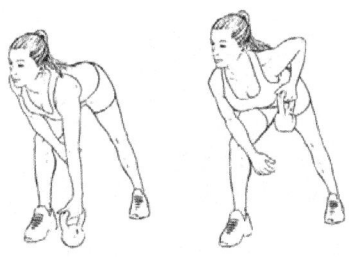

A single arm Kettlebell pulls

It is great for building a solid base and back.

Make sure to keep your back straight to avoid placing unnecessary tension onto your lower back.

Make sure you make sure you pull your shoulder back to maximize the benefits of the workout.

You should aim for 20 reps, 10 for each arm, and 3 sets.

Set a kettlebell up in the front of you

Put your right leg forward, and place your left foot on the heel of your left foot (similar to the lunge posture.)

Relax your knees as you bend them slightly to enter an upright position.

Make sure your back is straight.

Relax your right hand onto your right knee to provide security.

Take the kettlebell in your hands with a neutral grip the left side of your hand.

The kettlebell should be pulled up towards your stomach, then retracting your shoulder blade while stretching your elbow. Maintain your spine straight. Lower your body and repeat.

Perform all repetitions on one side prior to switching sides.

Pull-ups

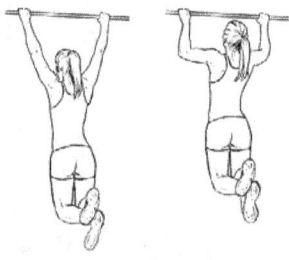

The classic move that can be modified from a tight grip to a wide grips to tackle different areas of the back.

Be sure to tighten your core when performing pull-ups, as it helps you to recruit additional muscles that will aid in your movement.

The towel could be draped over the bar, and then can be used to practice pull-ups before performing them to improve grip strength.

The knees can be elevated during pull-ups to strengthen the abdominal muscles.

You should aim for 20 reps, however in the case of a beginner, using a band or machine to increase your reps is recommended.

When you are standing under a pull-up bar, reach upwards and grasp the bar using your hands in an upward grip. Maintain your arms straight and stay atop the bar to ensure that your arms can take the entire weight.

Keep your body straight and not swaying your weight and pull your body upwards toward the bars by pulling the elbows downwards towards your torso in an angle.

Continue to lift to the point that your body is almost hitting the bar. You will feel an "squeeze" at the bottom of your lats (about halfway across your back, and towards your side) as they expand.

When your lats are fully stretched at the highest point of your movement gradually lower your body back to the starting position.

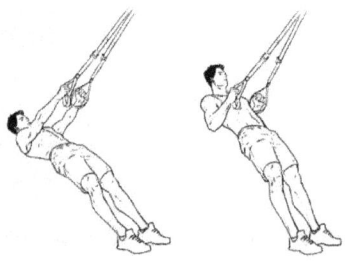

Suspension Strap Row

When you start to see reps that are easy, consider placing your feet on a swissball to make it harder and work your core.

Be sure to take your shoulders back to maximize the benefits of the movement.

Try to do 30 reps and three sets.

Grab the straps of suspension. As you stand with the straps in front then hold your lower back in place as well as your core.

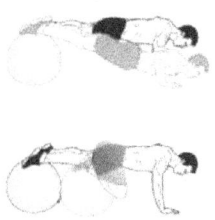

Lean back and let the straps support your weight. Your arms should be straight.

Lift yourself up using your back, while keeping a strong core.

Inhale the muscles of your back and slowly lower your body. Repeat.

If you are looking for more difficulty you can place a swissball the front of you and put your feet on top. Then, raise yourself to the point that you are able to balance yourself before completing the steps 1-4.

The Targeting of Your Chest

Kettlebell Swiss Ball Press

A great exercise to build your strength across various planes of motion, as well as building your core strength.

This movement also teaches both your arms and legs to work together, unlike the traditional bench press.

While you press the kettlebell, you want it to move up and down upon the Swiss ball, aiming to hit various directions of motion.

Aim for 30 x reps, 15 per side for 3 x sets.

Relax to the Swiss ball using kettlebells on to either on either side of your feet.

Hold both kettlebells with both hands and then bend them until the kettlebell's body is resting on your biceps.

The kettlebell should be pushed through until the full extend your arms.

Repeat on both sides to alter the range of movement.

Swiss-ball Pushup as well as Jackknife

Ideal for chest and core because it makes the push-up difficultdue to the incline angle and the balancing feature of the Swissball

Explore different ways to perform the exercise, such as using one leg for the swissball, or focusing on one leg for the pushup, making it more challenging.

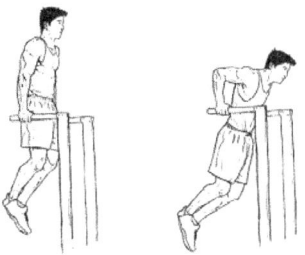

Try to do 15 reps per set for 3 sets.

Set your shins up on the Swiss ball and take an upright position with both hands straight with your arms spaced shoulder-width apart. This is the ideal starting point.

While keeping your body straight and straight, lower your body until it is almost touching the floor. Pause then push it back up as fast as you can.

Then, you roll the ball towards your chest, pulling it forward using both feet. Then, stop, and return to the original posture by dropping your hips, and rolling the ball backwards.

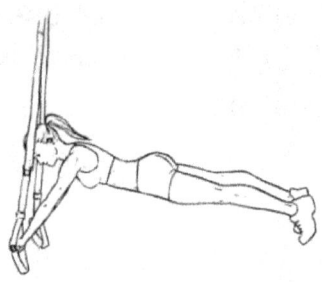

Tricep Dips

Try to get as deep as you can to get the maximum benefit of the dip.

Do not forget to lift knees during the move to provide an exercise that is a core exercise.

If you keep your spine straight with no leaning to the side, it will be able to work harder on your triceps.

If you're looking to strengthen the shoulders, then leaning to one side places the emphasis on your pecs.

Try to do 15 reps per set for 3 sets.

Take the dip bars in your hands with an overhand grip. Keep your elbows near to the body.

Allow your body weight to hang, so that it is supported by your shoulders and arms. Maintain your hips in a straight line.

Do the same thing with your palms. Push them down by lifting your arms. Lift your body to the point that your arms straight. (Do not lock your elbows.)

Reduce your body slowly by bend your elbows. Continue to lower your body downwards until you notice a slight stretch in your shoulders.

Pause and then return to your starting position.

Suspension Strap Press

Similar to the pull of the suspension strap this exercise is made more difficult by placing your feet on a swissball, which will help the core to participate in the exercise, and also to improve balance.

Make sure to work your way into the press, and then change the direction of your movement to engage more muscles during the workout.

Try to do 20 reps in 3 sets.

Place yourself in a position to push up using the straps to either the side of your arms.

Keep your feet beneath you as you hold the straps. Then walk back out again until you're in a standing position and with the straps in your hands.

Lower yourself , bracing your core, then push yourself back to the starting position.

Try placing a swissball underneath your feet to add more challenges.

Chapter 15: The Whole Body Exercises Or Holistic Workout

These types of exercises are what kettlebells were made to be used for. A majority of these workouts involve bodily movements that we perform every day, or are necessary to maintain the health and flexibility of the body. Therefore, the majority of these exercises must be performed with a certain amount of caution since having incorrect posture or form when performing them can panic to one kind of injury or an additional. If done in a safe way, they can be among the most enjoyable exercises you'll ever experience in your lifetime.

1. Russian Kettlebell Swing

Muscle group to target: Hips, Back, Shoulders, Legs, Glutes

Walkthrough The following is among the most simple, fundamental Kettlebell exercises you can do but it's also the most demanding. This Russian Kettlebell exercise is simple to master, simple to master and utilizes the entire physique from head to the toe. To master this technique simply stand up straight with your feet hips from each other and grasp the handle of the kettlebell while keeping your friends looking down as well as your hands straight. Lean your knees a bit and then push your hips back and lower your body slightly (not as far as you would do with an Squat). The kettlebell should be swung forward, stretching your legs and hips while you go. The weight is then lowered between your legs, completing one repetition.

When performing this exercise, it's crucial to remember that the primary movement is from your hips, not the arms, when you come back to an upright posture. If you do it correctly the exercise will work mostly your glutes, the lower back, core shoulders, arms and, of obviously your hips. This exercise can be completed in a single or two handed. If done using one hand, switch hands each time the kettlebell is in the starting place (between the legs) Remember that you should keep the free arm moving in a rhythmic manner to maintain the momentum.

2. the Sidestep Kettlebell Swing

Group of muscles to target: Legs, Glutes, and Back Shoulders, Glutes and Legs

Walkthrough: This workout is a variant of the workout described above. It has demonstrated that it's not just beneficial to add to any workout routine however, as there's lots of additional movement the exercise adds an additional experience that is viewed by many as thrilling. The majority of people are of the opinion that adding this variant to the swing of the kettlebell to your workout can help to break the monotony of your workout and can create a sense of excitement to your training environment.

To perform this exercise, you'll have to get the kettlebell in your hand and begin by swinging the kettlebell as that was described earlier. Once the kettlebell is between your feet, step left using your left foot. If the kettlebell is at its highest up in the sky, raise your left foot upwards to the right. Continue to sidestep in this way for the desired amount of repetitions. After the set then repeat the exercise but step side-stepping towards the reverse direction.

In the context of a set , this is a great exercise to attempt however why not test yourself to see how long it takes before giving up. This will let you know whether you're on the right course to meet your desired fitness level or if you need to work on your fitness.

3. It is the Kettlebell Lunge press

Muscle group to target: Shoulders Arms, Back, Legs, Glutes

Walkthrough Traditional lunges require simple, easy sequence of moves to achieve their aim. This routine promises to be a fascinating alternative to the standard lunge and is guaranteed to add a flavor to your exercise. In addition to focusing on your legs and glutes like traditional lunges it also aids in building your arms, shoulders and back muscles when pressing is included for a complete fitness routine.

Similar to the normal lunge, begin by standing upright and holding the kettlebell with one hand, at chest level with your elbow bent and your palm facing upwards. Sway forward using only one leg while lifting the kettlebell over your head. Reverse to the starting position and count the entire exercise in one repetition. After a certain number of repetitions change legs and hands, and repeat the exercise to complete a set.

This exercise is essential for people who want to increase strength in their legs and glutes. It is also extremely beneficial for those who want to build endurance and flexibility of their shoulders.

4. It's the Kettlebell Sumo High pull

The target muscle group is Shoulders, Arms Legs, Back, and Arms

Walkthrough The walkthrough is a fluid movement which can be used to improve back strength particularly for the lower back and is extremely efficient in helping you build strength and endurance in your legs. It can also be very effective in increasing muscle strength in the shoulders and arms.

For this exercise, you must first sit with the kettlebell in between your feet while keeping your feet slightly wider than your the distance between your shoulders. Relax into a standing position, while bending your knees slightly while pulling your hips back while keeping the back in a straight position. Take the kettlebell in both hands and raise it to your chin or shoulder height while you straighten your hips and legs. Bring the weight back down to the floor and between your legs for one repetition.

Rememberthat the primary for this exercise, like most exercises in the same location, is your hips. Although the arms have a role to play but this is only evident during the pulling phase towards the end when the kettlebell must get to shoulder height. While they play a small part, the advantages to your shoulders and arms after several sets of Sumo High Pull won't be missed.

Chapter 16: General Kettlebell Errors

We have previously discussed how kettlebell training can be efficient in increasing strength and strength. It's also evident that there's a broad variety of kettlebell-training tools that are available on the market, all of which play an important role. For example, the swing of the kettlebell is a key component in increasing the endurance of your body and also strengthens your posterior chain.

But, one thing you need to keep to keep in mind when you do kettlebell training it's not always enjoyable and fun. If you're just beginning it is essential that you keep an eye on what you're doing and how you're doing it in order to reduce the chance of injury.

If you're just beginning, ensure that you receive the instruction you require from a professional fitness trainer to guide you in learning to use kettlebells correctly. Here are a few most common errors to be aware of when using the kettlebell:

The first mistake is choosing A More Weight

For those who are just beginning, it can be extremely easy to get caught up in all the excitement and urge to go too far. The challenge is fun but it is important to be patient and take it slow to ensure that your body isn't in shock.

So instead of jumping into starting with heavy weights, it is recommended to start with the weights you are able to handle and move up gradually. If you are able to add the weight more than your body are able to take on, you'll restrict your movements in a bad way and increase the chance of sustaining an injury.

If you're training make sure that safety is your first priority. The best method to ensure this is to choose the appropriate weight for your kettlebell. Get advice from a professional when you choose which weights you will be using to begin your training. Make sure you're not mistaking the weights and measurements by understanding the distinction between centimeters and meters as well as kilograms and pounds.

The second error is that you generate force Through The Upper Part Of The Body

As we mentioned previously, kettlebell exercises typically involve moves of the whole body. This is what makes exercises twice as efficient. There are many beginners level that try to get stronger through these exercises. It is essential to recognize that this could put excessive strain over your body's upper part, and be careful not to do it.

Misstake 3: Swinging The Kettlebell too fast

A crucial thing you need to be aware of is that if you use the kettlebell too quickly it is possible to lose control and pulling on your muscles, which could cause serious injuries. While it's enjoyable to lift the kettlebell with such force following a long day, there's the possibility that it could cause more harm than good when your posture is weakened.

The 4th Mistake: Focusing On Quantity

If you are a novice you have a good likelihood that you'll be tempted to overdo it and work yourself too hard. If your instructor suggests starting with ten reps, but you want to go higher than that may not be an ideal idea.

I guarantee you that finishing 20 reps in a poor technique is worse than never lifting kettlebells because you're employing the wrong method. It is vital to do each kettlebell exercise the way it should be done so that you don't suffer from the negative consequences that could result in injuries. Be sure to follow the rules before you attempt to do any exercise.

5. Mistake: Putting on the Wrong Running Shoes

As I said earlier, the best part is that you don't need to put on a specific kind of shoe to perform this workout. However, this doesn't mean that you cannot wear shoes that put the risk of injuries.

Although it can be tempting to put on shoes with extremely large soles, you have to be aware that this could slow your movement when working out.

When you are doing kettlebell exercises, it's recommended to wear shoes that let you naturally move your ankles as well as lower leg ligaments and your feet. Running shoes that are thick do not just cushion

The heels can also cause to elevate the heel off the ground and cause that your foot's grip to become weak.

Chapter 17: What Much Are You Capable To Lift?

The most important concerns to consider when you're training using kettlebells, particularly if you're starting out from scratch to train, is how much weight can you handle? As previously mentioned, proper technique is essential to ensure safe and efficient kettlebell training . And since it requires unique dynamic movements which include high-intensity interval work making sure you are able to apply the correct quantity of weight is vital.

For a beginner, it's important to have to pay to selecting the correct weight for your kettlebell exercise program. The process of selecting the ideal kettlebell weight can be difficult, especially when you've never attempted any kind of weight-training prior to now. It's possible to feel that the lightest kettlebell weight can be too heavy.

However it is possible that it's been some time, but using traditional items of equipment such as dumbbells and barbells as well as suspension trainers. There's a chance you'll find that what I suggest might be "nothing other than the size of a small amount of peanuts" according to your own perception. In this case I'll have to ask to temporarily suspend your beliefs regarding resistance or weight training and instead, consider kettlebells with a new and different angle. If you don't, you'll be having difficulty understanding what kettlebell training actually is, and will consequently are more likely to have difficulty having that body you've been imagining.

It's crucial that as you are learning how to train using kettlebells, you follow the guidelines that almost all trainers across the world expect of their students: keep an open-minded mind be attentive, and take notes. While I am sure you'll be able to learn a lot from this book that you can begin working with kettlebells in the future I would still strongly suggest you to attend at least one exercise session under the guidance of a qualified kettlebell instructor to avoid injury risk by through proper form and maximising the muscle-building and fat-burning effects that the exercise will bring.

Be aware that kettlebell training isn't exactly the equivalent to isolated training using weights. A lot of kettlebell-related exercises are compound, i.e., involves several muscles. Furthermore, a lot of these exercises are full body and involve "throwing" your kettlebells about. You're probably not familiar with this kind of workout before so it's essential to start by keeping an open-mind, and resist the temptation to think that there's not new.

The minimum amount of training couple of sessions with a professional kettlebell instructor will allow you to master the basics but more complicated moves. No amount of books or videos can ever come close to the level of precise feedback and attention to detail that a couple of sessions with a kettlebell expert can provide. This feedback will aid you in maximizing the benefits of body-shredding and decrease the risk of injury during kettlebell training.

If you do kettlebell exercises in a good technique, you'll be able to enhance your ability to control your body. You'll also be able to drastically reducing your time for workouts and accomplish your goals, including getting shredded! In addition to getting your body shredded, you'll be able do it without boredom! It's a win-win I guess?

From various core movements kettlebell exercises have developed into a myriad of innovative and thrilling techniques and movements. Like the slogan from one of the most loved junk food go the moment you begin the kettlebell, you'll never stop. In fact, you probably will not wish to.

Now we return to the question of how much weight should you be lifting?

For Men

For men, a great starting weight for most workouts is 16 kilograms which is 35 pounds. If you're a man and you're wondering, "35 pounds is peanuts when compared to my 100-pound bench press!" Hold on for one minute, Sparky! Although 35 pounds might be an unassuming barbell or dumbbell weight, it's definitely not the light kettlebell weight! Rememberthat kettlebells come with distinctive handles and shapes!

If you take a look 35 pounds could not be much to perform deadlifts, squats or even curls of the barbell! However, since you're not doing these particular exercises at least not using the barbell, 35 pounds could actually be more powerful than what you can get through barbells. This is due to the particular way kettlebells are used to perform exercises.

You'll likely be able activate a variety of muscles that you're not capable of doing with traditional exercises for weights or resistance and equipment. It's possible to awaken several muscles that are "sleeping" muscles. And believe me when I say that many of your muscle groups (upper lower legs, the abs along with the lower back) will feel like they're burning up in the first or two. This is due to the fact that kettlebell training typically involves intense interval workouts, i.e., brief but extremely intense stretching exercises with the least amount of time between sets.

Based on the above, you'll have to select a moderately small weight, in relation to the kettlebell experience you've had beginning that is around 35 pounds for a man. If you feel it's too heavy, try the kettlebell with a lighter weight and if you think it's too light, you can adjust it according to your needs.

However, don't think you can consider a 35-pound, 16-kg kettlebell for granted! Many people who are new to kettlebell instruction are at risk of not executing the correct form when exercising with kettlebells by muscle-stretching or powering through the exercises. What's the reason? The reason is because they're using kettlebells that are not their ability to lift them using the proper technique. Is it because of their ego? Perhaps.

A 35-pound kettlebell is sufficient for males who are just beginning to exercise in a the correct posture. As I've already mentioned you can alter the weight accordingly with a higher kettlebell that is weighted.

For Women

If you're a female the ideal starting weight is an 18-pound kettlebell, or an 8-kilogram one. Like the kettlebell that weighs 35 pounds for males, this one is a middle weight that's ideal to begin kettlebell training with.

When you first take the kettlebell weighing 18 pounds and attempt to complete a single-arm, upright row naturally (i.e. without regard of proper lifting form) it's easy to think "Wow that was simple. What's the reason the author suggested that I begin using this particular size?" But as I previously mentioned for men that a "lighter" weight could appear to be much, more hefty when you train with kettlebells due to the distinctive design and shape. Its unique shape can change the bicep curl with a dumbbell, which is an isolation workout to a more complicated one when it is done using kettlebells.

If you practice kettlebell exercises in a proper way it will allow you to build your body for greater control of your body as well as reduce the time you'll need to put out every session to be shredder, and accomplish your goals, both functional and attractive (i.e. an energised body). Through kettlebell-based exercises, the majority of your lifting will not only involve your arm or leg as well, but your entire core as well as your entire upper and lower body.

A warning for both men and women

Many believe that selecting the wrong weight for your work is working with a load that is too heavy. It is also possible to choose the wrong weight if you are lifting too much. What is the reason why lifting too light a mistake?

Remember the importance of proper or good form? Then, lifting a light weight has a an increased risk of only exercising your muscles, or pushing with ballistic movements rather than following the correct form, which could be more difficult, but also stimulating your muscles. If this happens, the most likely you'll be throwing weights about - without concern for proper form like they're made from paper. If you continue to adhere to poor shape, the less you'll be able make gains in regards to weight and strength, muscle strength and cutting down body fat. So, avoid the lure to believe that light is the best. Do not believe that light is right... It's right!

The Pood

There's no way to tell if it's an electronic tablet made by an electronics manufacturer whose name comes from a fruit, which symbolizes the lure. If you're asked "What is the pood of your kettlebell?" they're simply asking you how heavy the kettlebell that you're using.

Also "pood "pood" is an Russian measurement of weight. If you thought there was just one system of measuring, which is the American and British methods of measuring Here comes the Russians to create further confusion!

A pood equivalent to around 16 kilograms which is 36 pounds. If you're interested in Crossfit and begin to learn about kettlebells you'll hear about this measure more frequently.

How to Choose the Best Kettlebell

In addition to picking the ideal kettlebell weight, it is essential to be able to select an excellent kettlebell. Its quality can influence the ability of you to train with kettlebells effectively, so make sure you choose carefully. Here are some good tips to select a top kettlebell:

Select a kettlebell with an outer coating that is chip-resistant and smooth to ensure that your hands aren't easily inflamed, particularly when you perform stamina-building workouts for long durations of time. A good kettlebell has sleek and curved handles that can be easily gripped from any angle of the handle, not only at the top.

A top kettlebell provides enough space between its handle and kettlebell to ensure maximum bone stacking during press and lifts with snatch. The shape of the handle is also required to enable you to grasp the edges of the handle - sometimes referred to as horns - to perform specific exercises. The coating of the handle must match the kettlebell's, and be smooth, so that you can minimize the chance of scratches, blisters or cuts on your fingers.

The best kettlebells are non-rust and protected by a lifetime warranty .

A further characteristic of a kettlebell that is of high-quality are high-contrast fonts that enable you to quickly identify the kettlebell you're planning to utilize.

Finally, a good quality kettlebell should be one that is comfortable to hold. Factors that could impact your ability to hold your kettlebell are the width and the diameter of the handles and the distance between the upper part of the handle and handle's bottom and the overall diameter of the bell.

Once you're ready to train with kettlebells Let's move on to the exercises or workouts in themselves. The exercises are divided into three sections - each one for upper body the lower part of the body and the combination or total body exercises. The most important thing to achieve your body that is ripped is to exercise every week 3 times for 20-30 minutes in a row, with little rest between sets. By minimal, I mean not greater than 30 secs between each set. Try to do at least three sets for each exercise, and, of course, maintain perfect form all the time.

Chapter 18: A Guide To Kettlebell And Crossfit Instruction

Due to the flexibility of kettlebells that can be used in the training routine of every athlete, it is frequently employed in the training regimen for CrossFit practitioners. The people who employ this equipment in their CrossFit training programs usually focus on building endurance and strength.

If you're unfamiliar with CrossFit it is a well-known training and strength program that is used in gyms around the globe. The program is designed to enhance your overall fitness by implementing the use of high-intensity exercises. The three major kinds of exercises you'll encounter in CrossFit include gymnastics, aerobics and Olympic weight-lifting exercises. The workouts you perform will change every day. Certain CrossFit gyms also have programs specifically for people with physical requirements, such as martial arts, sports training, or professional fitness.

A typical CrossFit session will consist of an assortment of warm-up exercises followed by a skill-building exercise. Then it's time for you will be working on the Workout of the Day or the WoD will be followed by the Workout of the Day. Each gym has its individual workout plan for the day, but there are some that adhere to the routine of the day recommended through the CrossFit website. The workout usually concludes by stretching exercises to reduce the stress on muscles. There are gyms that focus their WoDs on increasing the strength, similar to Olympic Weight lifting.

Following the workout your performance at completing your workout will be evaluated and with other participants you workout with. Some people also schedule their exercise sessions. This can make the gym environment even more fiercely competitive.

Using Kettlebells

For fitness enthusiasts with only a few workout tools at home, executing the routine of the day won't produce results due to the need for tools needed to complete specific tasks. This is where kettlebells is a great option. Instead of adhering to the WoD on the CrossFit website or nearby gym, you can begin practicing CrossFit at home using kettlebells. It is possible to do this doing the kettlebell workouts that are included within this publication.

This is less expensive than joining the gym. It's also more practical than following the recommended exercise of the day on the CrossFit website. It's also an excellent alternative for those who aren't confident that they can complete just one CrossFit session.

Utilizing the 30-day cycle

In the next chapter, you'll follow a 30-day program with kettlebells only. A month of exercise routine based on these suggestions will help you build up enough muscles and endurance to help prepare you for more CrossFit exercises.

It is also recommended that you exercise with a buddy or family member. In addition to the intense exercises, the success of CrossFit is largely because of the community that supports it. Be sure to become part of the local CrossFit communities within your area. There are a few of them at local gyms and clubs. The social aspect of the community can not only increase your level of competition, but also serves as an excellent source of information and suggestions to help you improve your performance.

Chapter 19: The Most Capable Soviet Kettlebell Routines

We'll provide you with training programs that are geared at two distinct training objectives:

Fat Loss

Muscle Gain

Three workouts will be provided to accomplish each goal which will enable you to advance your training from a beginner level to an advanced levels.

The Tabata Protocol

The Fat Loss exercises will include a high-quality cardio routine which will boost your fat loss to a new level. It's known as Tabata Protocol. Tabata Protocol

Tabata Protocol Tabata Protocol all began with the Japanese Olympic Speed Skating Team. The head coach, Irisawa Koichi, created an high intensity Interval Training workout to his team of skaters. The workout consisted of eight rounds. Each round took just 20 minutes of hard training with a cycling ergometer. This was and then 10 seconds of relaxation. Koichi has one of his trainers, Azumi Tabata, analyze the effectiveness of the exercise by using techniques that are scientific. This is how it was that the Tabata Protocol (which HIIT training is based on) emerged. Tabata wasn't the one who invented the technique of training but due to the huge attention to his findings, the workout was named for his name. Tabata's research revealed that his subjects with impressive results, which render traditional (steady steady state) cardio seem uneffective in the comparison.

To complete Tabata Protocol, you must follow the Tabata Protocol with Kettlebells simply perform the move for 20 minutes and then take 10 seconds timer. Repeat for the set amount of sets.

The Fat Loss Exercise

Beginning Workout for Fat Loss

Warm-Up

Around-the-body-pass : 30 s each direction using a kettlebell with a light weight.

Halo : 30 seconds each direction, using a kettlebell with a light weight.

Kettlebell deadlift: 10 reps

Goblet squat: 10 reps

Workout

Two-handed Kettlebell Swing Tabata Protocol for 20 seconds with 10 seconds of rest between arms. Repeat 4 times with one minute recovery between sets.

Single Press Tabata procedure for 20 minutes with a rest of 10 seconds before switching arms. Repeat for 4 sets , with 1 minute recovery between sets.

Warm-Down

Jogging for 10 minutes is easy.

Five minutes of stretching 30 sec per side, for every stretch (behind-the-back shoulder stretch; shoulder stretch the triceps pulls; standing knee-to chest stretch and standing quadriceps stretch

Intermediate Workout to Lose Fat

Warm-Up

Single-leg kettlebell deadlift 8 reps per side

Windmill: 10 reps on each side

Joint mobility exercises: Rotate the major joints (shoulders the hips, neck) 10-15 times.

Workout

Complete the most rounds you can within 10 minutes:

Double swing: 15 reps with kettlebells that are medium-weight

Double Clean : 15 reps with kettlebells that are medium-weight

Double front squat: 15 reps using kettlebells of medium weight

Russian twist: 40 twists using kettlebells of medium-weight

Warm-Down

Jogging for 10 minutes is easy.

Five minutes of stretching 30 sec per side, for every stretch (behind-the-back shoulder stretch; shoulder stretch pulling triceps muscles, standing knee-to-chest stretch (pg. standing quadriceps stretch

Advanced Workout to Lose Fat

Warm-Up

Jogging for 5 minutes is easy.

Dynamic mobility exercises: arm twists both forward and backwards for 30s and clapping dynamically for 30 seconds, leg swings in all directions for 30 seconds

Workout

Goblet Squat : 30 s each side

The flexion of the spine : Hold for 1 minute

Calf stretch : 1 min per leg

Two-Arm Kettlebell Row Tabata Protocol for 20 minutes with a 10 second rest. Repeat for 4 sets.

Lunge Clean/Lunge press: Tabata method for 20 seconds with a rest of 10 seconds. Repeat for 4 sets.

Static stretches: 30 seconds each side , or 10 reps for each practice (standing quadriceps stretch stretching hamstrings standing and a standing knee-to-chest stretch stretching the calf; spinal flexion)

It is the Muscle Gain Workouts

Beginning Workout for Muscle Gain

Jogging for 5 minutes is easy.

Joint mobility exercises The key to joint mobility is to rotate the major joints (shoulders and hips, neck,) 10-20 times for 5 minutes.

Perform 10 repetitions of each of the listed exercises on the opposite side of your body. Do not stop. Repeat 3 times, taking one minute of time in between rounds. The first round comprises of a single swing, one cleanse, one press the snatch the goblet and squat.

Stretch for 7 minutes Each stretch should be performed for 1 minute (behind-the-back shoulder stretch standing knee-to-chest stretch stretching hamstrings in a standing position and standing quadriceps stretch and the child's pose; spinal extension and the flexion of your spine).

Intermediate Training for Muscle Gain

Warm-Up

Jogging for 5 minutes is easy.

Body-weight squat: 1 set for 30 s

Mobility exercises for joints: 20 repetitions from each (hip circles and torn trunks, bends in the lateral shoulder rolls, waist bends neck tiltsand turns, the ankle bounce).

Workout

Rack hold For 2 minutes: hold with two kettlebells of light weight Rest 1 minute Hold for 2 min using two kettlebells of moderate weight Rest for 2 minutes Hold for one minute using two kettlebells that weigh a lot.

Overhead hold: hold 1 minute using two kettlebells Rest for 1 minute then hold for 1 min using two kettlebells with moderate weights.

Single Arm Press Perform two sets with 5 repetitions for each hand, and rest for 1 minute between sets.

Two-Arm Kettlebell Rows: Perform three sets with 10 repetitions each, resting for 1 minute between sets.

Russian Twist: Perform three sets with 15 reps each, taking a break of 1 minute between each set.

Farmer's Carry: Use two kettlebells that are heavy for as long as is possible for one set.

Warm-Down

Jogging for 5 minutes is easy.

Stretch for 7 mins Each stretch should be performed for 1 minute (behind-the-back shoulder stretch standing knee-to-chest stretch stretching hamstrings in a standing position and standing quadriceps stretch with spine extension; child's posture and the flexion of your spine).

Advanced Training for Muscle Gain

Warm-Up

Squats with body weight 30 reps for 1 set.

Skip rope: 1 minute

Active mobility with dynamic motion: 15 repetitions of each arm to both directions, chest to hollow and expand; chest vertical opening; dynamic clapping leg swings

Workout

Turkish Get-up 5 reps per arm

Goblet Squat 5 sets , 5 reps taking a break for 1 minute between sets

One Arm Cleansing: 1 minute and rest for 1 minute

Snatch: 1 minute and rest for 1 minute

High Pull High Pull: Five sets of 10 reps taking a break of 1 minute between sets

Warm-Down

Jogging for 10 minutes is easy.

Stretch for 7 minutes Do each stretch for one minute (behind-the-back shoulder stretch stretching with knees in a standing position; stretching hamstrings in a standing position stretching the quadriceps in a standing position with spine extension; child's posture and the flexion of your spine).

Chapter 20: The Heart Rate

How can you determine the Heart Rate?

It is crucial for a person to determine the heart rate since an unusually low or high could indicate a health issue. This is why it is the easy method to determine the heart rate is through a pulses, which are typical, is located in the wrist, inside the elbow, the back of the neck and the top part of your foot. There are a few steps to help you calculate the heart rate accurately:

1. The first step is to ease your body and locate an area that is comfortable. It is essential that a person isn't in a state of trance and remains motionless for minimum five to 10 minutes.

Step 2: When the body is relaxed, locate the radial artery , or pulse at the appropriate location and apply pressure using your middle or index fingers.

Step 3: Once you have completed this, you should count how many beats that an individual feels for ten seconds using the digital watch.

Fourth step: The procedure must be repeated three to four times to get the exact heart rate and determine the average. Then multiply the result by six to get the RHR.

5. It is important to keep a regular check to on track and ensure that a healthy RHR has been maintained.

If your resting heart rate remains consistently higher than 100, then it is crucial to talk with an experienced doctor in order to avoid serious issue. Additionally, if a person does not engage in intense physical activity like professional athletes, it could be an indication of a health issue. Particularly, if someone experiences constant dizziness shortness of breath, or even fainting. In contrast, studies show the possibility that having a rate lower 60 could result from the use of medications. Additionally, athletes or people who exercise regularly tend to have lower heart rates since their muscles are effective and in good shape and require less effort. A person who is less active or who lives a more habit of sitting may be able to have a heart rate that is between 60 and 100 because the muscles are required to work harder to sustain bodily functions.

Target Heart Rates

Many factors affect the heart rate including poor eating habits, inactivity and unhealthy lifestyle habits like excessive use of tobacco or drugs. In addition, the rate of heart beat is also affected by the overall health and fitness of the person. Beyond that, researches suggest that age is an important factor in affecting the heart rate since young hearts work faster and more effectively than those who are beyond 60.

It is recommended that you track your heart rate to reap benefits and enhance your the condition of your heart. The ideal heart rate zone is somewhere between 50 between 85 and 50 percent their max heart rate. The most popular method to determine this is to subtract the age of your child from 220. For instance, a person who is 30, is able to subtract 220 and will get an average of 190. The ideal zone for a person who is 30 years old is between 50 and 85 percent of his maximum heart rate, so multiply the numbers 190 x 0.50 and 191 0.50 x 0.85 that will give 95 bpm and 162 BPM and 162 bpm, respectively. For people older than 40, they should subtract 10.75 multiplied by age from the formula because it may underestimate the heart rate at which you are most comfortable.

Additionally, adults of age can help compensate for slow heart through making use out of every beat. A larger, stronger heart can compensate for a slower rate by pumping more blood every time it beats. The aim of exercise in older people

Alter Target HR Zone, 50-85% average Maximum Heart Rate 100 percent

20 years 100-180 beats per minute . 200 beats per min.

30 years, 95-162 beats per minute. Minute 190 beats per minute.

35 years 93-157 beats/minute 35 years 185 beats a minute

60 years 90-153 beats/ hour 180 beats per minute

45 years 88-149 beats a minutes 175 beats

50 years 85-145 beats a Minute 170 beats/minute

55 years 83-140 beats a minute 165 beats/minute

60 years of age 80-136 beats a Minute 160 beats per

65 years 78-132 beats/minute 15 beats per minute

70 years 75-28 beats/minute 150 beats/minute

Chapter 21: Widen Your Legs And Warming Up

I'm not trying being one of these people However, what you've been taught about stretching isn't true.

It's possible to think that each workout begins by using a butterfly, rubbing your toes, and performing an extension of your leg, as you did when you were in gym class as a kid. However, recent research suggests there isn't the best method to prepare your body to exercise. Instead, you should make it a habit to do light exercises to warm your muscles and joints and start to generate heat to your body, to the point where you're breaking into a light sweat. The static stretching method doesn't accomplish this, but active exercises that are full body and gentle work do.

A different method

Instead of this traditional, stretch-before-you-train model, I will make 3 simple suggestions of how to structure your mobility routine. What we're looking for is an entire system of stability and mobility. If you're looking to gain a good understanding of this, you should read Becoming a Supple Leopard or The Roll Model

1. Dynamic movements using a single stretch

2. Morning or nighttime stretching

3. Single ankle and single arm strength exercises

Dynamic movement

Dynamic movement is a method to stretch joints and muscles prior to an intense exercise. In contrast to static stretching an active warm-up involves full-body exercises. I typically start at on top, and gradually work my way downwards.

Neck rotations

Arm circles

Arm is swung

Arms of the cross body swing

Band pass-through

Trunk rotation

Hip circles

Leg turns

Leg swings from side to side

Ankle circles

Air squats

I'll typically continue with something similar to:

4 minutes of jumping rope

or

800 meter run

or

For 4 minutes, row

Stretching and mobility

The act of stretching is something you should to become habitual of doing for hours ahead or right after you have worked out. The practice of stretching prior to a workout has been proven to not improve performance in any way, and new research has suggested that stretching before an exercise can actually result in a negative impact on overall performance.

One of my favorite ways to relax is rooted in the yin yoga. Yin is a type of yoga that I've been practicing for nearly 8 years . It is a form of yoga where you do static postures for between 2 and 5 minutes while breathing deeply breathing patterns, which are rhythmic. Based on what I've observed, it's one of the most effective methods to relax the body, strengthen weak muscles, ease tension (which is essential during a prolonged block of exercise) and to develop creative mobility.

Find online the yin yoga routines and if you're looking to get an excellent paid online service that will guide you through your stretching routine, I can't be more pleased to recommend www.romwod.com enough. You can also use straps and stretch bands to enhance the effectiveness of your stretching routine.

Another approach to create mobility is by releasing tight muscles and sore muscles through the help of massage rollers, foam rollers balls and sticks. This is a sophisticated method and I suggest buying and reading a book such as Becoming a Supple Leopard or The Roll Model to give yourself a clear understanding of how this works.

For night time foam rolling session, I'll usually use a method like:

2.30 minutes rolling each of the feet the ball of lacrosse

3 minutes of attacking each leg using a foam roller

2 minutes devoted to stretching my neck and back

2 minutes for each hip using a lacrosse or kinesio balls

The routine of 9-10 minutes will loosen tight muscles, loosen my neck and spine as well as move blood to assist me in recovering from my the training.

Stability training

Stability refers to the capacity to stay in one place and not move when needed.

The requirements of an obstacle course mean that stability is of most crucial importance. There are many small connective tissues and muscles that lung to general stability. They are able to be trained in the same way as larger muscles. Below is an example exercise that can be utilized to increase stability and single leg mobility.

1. 4 10 single leg deadlift (using kettlebells or dumbbells)

2. Single arm snatching overhead squat (using kettlebell or dumbbell)

3. Single leg 4x8 Band assisted or TRX pistols

4. One minute of warrior poses with each foot for three times

5. One minute plank side for 3 rounds

Another fantastic way to increase stability is by using one of the agility ladders. Check out agility ladder exercises on YouTube and you'll discover some amazing examples of how you can integrate it into the training. It's a fantastic warm-up tool, and it's not even the most difficult!

When you combine all of these elements by combining all of these pieces, you can improve your body's durability and free of injuries, and fully recuperated.

Off days

Off days are just as important like training day, but you can't think of training all day without breaks - this could determined to overtraining injuries and injury from overuse. However, these days off are still an essential component of your training, when you utilize them properly.

The days off are the perfect time to work on the exercises for mobility we discussed earlier. Do yoga for an hour or stretching for 30 minutes and rolling.

If not, take the time now to organize and prepare your meals to ensure that you're eating healthy and nutritious food throughout the week. If you're feeling extremely exhausted you can go for a lengthy stroll, relax and perhaps think about making things using your hands.

Make time to plan your training time and create a schedule for your training.

The most important thing to remember is that there aren't any off days however this doesn't mean that you need to be a slug all week long. Simply make your days off just as effective as training day.

Conclusion

Kettlebells have been used for longer than we think, and they're not new and have an exciting opportunity ahead in the realm of competitive and fitness. Since kettlebells have become the most popular item in fitness and gyms and fitness studios, so are women discovering the benefits of strengthening.

The days when women shied away from work; now we take up the task and show guys who's the boss. All over the world, women are doing it, and you could too. The most appealing thing is that you won't only shed weight when you train with kettlebells but also have a lot of enjoyment!

Kettlebells are becoming more popular for women looking to be strong, slim and fit and it's not surprising why. They're extremely versatileand offer an entire set of powerful exercises to fight the fat. They've been known to be effective in reducing fat that can burn up to 400 calories in 20 minutes, and exercising up to 600 muscles in one exercise. There's no other exercise tool that gives you this versatility, with a small amount of time and space, and at the price of a reasonable one.

The use of kettlebells can provide you with intense workouts that require only a brief period of time with the highest fat burning benefits. They're compact, needing minimal space to work in and are also portable, meaning they can be taken anywhere and work out anytime. You don't have to visit the gym, and you can train in the comfort at your home. Kettlebells provide you with no reason to put off a workout or put off getting started.

This is your opportunity to make a positive difference to your life, a change that you can make for yourself as well as an investment in your self. If you choose to purchase kettlebells, you're creating a lifetime love affair with your fitness, health and your body. Whatever your goals may be kettlebells will assist you to reach them and help you appear attractive while you go. The age-old tools for strength training have altered not only my own life, but those of thousands of women all over the globe who have embraced their glow. Now , you can transform your life as well with the advice I've shared in this book to begin your journey towards a more positive and healthier you.

Thank you for giving me the opportunity to share my knowledge and passion with you. I'm ecstatic that you've spent the time reading this book, which was written by me as a way of helping you achieve your weight reduction goals. It's time to begin looking for your next favorite companion, a kettlebell that is brand new, and begin your journey now.